# Bodily Harm

## Symphysiotomy and Pubiotomy in Ireland 1944–92

### *Marie O'Connor*

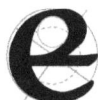

evertype
2011

Published by Evertype, 19A Corso Street, Dundee, DD2 1DR, Scotland. www.evertype.com.

First edition 2011. Reprinted with corrections October 2024.

A catalogue record for this book is available from the British Library.

ISBN-10 1-904808-75-1
ISBN-13 978-1-904808-75-6

Typeset in Warnock Pro by Valerie Seery.

Cover: Michael Everson after Valerie Seery.

# Contents

*This report is dedicated to survivors of symphysiotomy in Ireland, Africa, India, Papua New Guinea and other far flung places.*

# Foreword

Shortly after writing an opinion piece for the *Sunday Independent* on the practice of 'Caesarean hysterectomy' at the Lourdes Hospital in September 2008,[1] I received a telephone call from a survivor of symphysiotomy: a meeting with three casualties of this operation followed. I had a background in policy-oriented research and a special interest in obstetrics, having been commissioned by the Department of Health to do a national survey on intentional home birth.[2] My first book documented women's experiences of maternity care[3], while my most recent one explained why our health system is as it is.[4] So believing that I could make some contribution to survivors' long running quest for justice, I agreed to see if I could help.

Survivors of Symphysiotomy (SoS) is a remarkable organisation by any standards. Dotted all over Ireland, members range in age from the late 50s to the late 80s. The sole dedicated voice of survivors in Ireland, SoS has been trying to secure an independent inquiry into the surgery for almost a decade. All such attempts have been thwarted. Founding members, such as Rose Magee, did not live to see the day. Despite the promises made to her by a former Minister for Health, the failure of Dublin City Council to install a stair lift left Rose a prisoner in her own home during her last years. Other indomitable founding members, such as Matilda Behan, Eileen Murphy and Claire Kavanagh — some now well into their 80s — continue to fly the flag. The courage, tenacity and determination of SoS members has been an unfailing inspiration to me in preparing this report. For very many of them, symphysiotomy has been a life sentence without remission.

---

[1]  Marie O'Connor 2008 'Mutilated by brutal 'surgery of last resort'.' *Sunday Independent* 7 Sept.

[2]  Marie O'Connor 1992. *Women and Birth: a national study of intentional home births in Ireland.* Unpublished Report for the Department of Health and Children.

[3]  Marie O'Connor 1995 *Birth Tides: turning towards home birth.* Pandora, London.

[4]  Marie O'Connor 2007 *Emergency: Irish hospitals in chaos.* Gill and Macmillan, Dublin.

It has taken me nearly three years of research to understand this childbirth surgery in all of its dreadful dimensions. Doctors described symphysiotomy as 'widening the pelvis', a benign description that obscured the fact that the surgery severed the pelvis, and one that had made its way into the media. The fact that symphysiotomy was carried out by doctors as a matter of personal preference meant that Caesarean section — the treatment of choice for obstructed labour at that time — was being withheld from the patient. Doctors also performed a related operation, cutting the pubic bone rather than the joint of the *symphysis pubis*. This operation, known as pubiotomy, was even more dangerous than symphysiotomy. I was also to learn that the operation posed significant risks to babies as well as mothers: medical evidence suggests that one baby in ten did not survive the operation of symphysiotomy, and survivor testimony shows one baby born in this way suffered catastrophic injuries.

Some symphysiotomies, particularly those performed in the aftermath of a Caesarean section, were more hideous than others. Those carried out during late pregnancy were almost equally unprecedented. However, even the more usual symphysiotomies, those done during labour, were cruel in the extreme. Women found the experience utterly traumatising: after being left in labour for many hours, they were generally operated upon without warning, in the labour ward or in theatre, under local anaesthetic. And after the surgery, there was still a baby to be born: they were still in labour.

The pain of pushing a baby out with an unhinged pelvis was followed by the agony of walking on it. Instead of immobilising the pelvis, hospital staff further destabilised it by requiring women to walk. Discharged home with a broken pelvis, women were left to sink or swim, without medical advice or painkillers. Many of the serious health problems — of mobility, pain and incontinence — endured by women today are related to the negligent failure to treat them as surgical patients.

In addition to medical negligence, there were other issues, such as the use, or abuse, of medical power and knowledge. The idea that major surgery could be performed on a pivotal structure of the body without patient consent was troubling enough. I knew that women were generally not informed in advance about their surgery, that the its risks and benefits had not been explained, nor the existence of a safer alternative, Caesarean section, mentioned. The failure of hospital staff to inform women of their surgery postnatally was even more disturbing, however. Even general practitioners refused, on occasion, to tell women what had been done to them.

Several decades were to elapse before many women finally understood that their pelvises had been broken. It was as though these were secret operations, not to be disclosed to the patient. Was it because the surgery was so aberrant that it could not be revealed?

Finally, there was the discovery that symphysiotomy is now enjoying a revival in resource poor countries, where it is promoted by some as a 'safe', low cost alternative to Caesarean section. However, as the lived experience of survivors shows and medical writings attest, the safety of symphysiotomy is a fallacy.

*Bodily Harm* examines in detail how the authorities in Ireland have dealt with demands for truth, justice, health and disability services since the surgery was first exposed in the media by Dr Jacqueline Morrissey in 1999. The report sets out the history of symphysiotomy and pubiotomy, describes how these operations were revived in an era when women in Ireland had few rights, and scrutinises the various claims that have been made for the surgery. In the closing chapters, I look at these operations from a legal perspective, show how the surgery was driven by medical ambition as well as religious beliefs and present survivors' case for truth and justice.

A word on the text. Throughout this report, I have sought to highlight and refute the myths and red herrings emanating from the specialty, both individually, and collectively (by the Institute of Obstetricians and Gynaecologists). Some of these statements appear in text panels. Except where otherwise stated, names and other identifying details have been changed to preserve womens' anonymity. Quoted statements are from survivors' written testimony, formal interviews and personal communication. All references to symphysiotomy in this report include pubiotomy unless otherwise indicated, as 'symphysiotomy' was used indiscriminately to denote pubiotomy in hospital clinical reports.[5]

Like historian Dr Frances Finnegan, whose work on the Magdalen Asylums[6] is as inspiring as it is meticulous, I do not think it a virtue to suspend one's moral judgement. I have sought to bring a view to the latter day practice of symphysiotomy in Ireland that is wider than medicine, one that encompasses feminist, sociological, legal, historical and midwifery perspectives. Some of the issues raised, however, such as the role of medicine in our society, are so wide ranging as to lie outside the parameters of this report. While this report is dedicated to survivors, none have sought in any way to influence its contents, nor should they be take as reflecting the views of SoS as a voluntary organisation.

While any errors in this report are my own, I should like to thank certain individuals and organisations. My thanks to my expert readers, Mavis Kirkham, Emeritus Professor of Midwifery at Sheffield Hallam University, whose crystal-clear insights into clinical matters deepened my understanding of these operations; and to Dr Janette Allotye, a medical historian with a special interest in the history of the pelvis, whose detailed reading of my work was invaluable. Michael Lynn, barrister-at-law at the Irish Bar and an expert in patient human rights, contributed significantly to the legal chapter. Dr Jacqueline Morrissey, a historian with a special interest in the influence of religious beliefs on clinical practice, was extremely generous with her work, which threw new light on the historical record, illuminating the fine, if occasionally shocking, detail of clinical practice. My gratitude, also, goes to SoS's

---

[5]   'National Maternity Hospital Report 1950' *Irish Journal of Medical Science* 1951: 832. In Jacqueline K Morrisey 2004 *An examination of the relationship between the Catholic Church and the medical profession in Ireland in the period 1922 – 1992, with particular emphasis on the impact of this relationship in the field of reproductive medicine.* Unpublished PhD thesis University College Dublin, 177.

[6]   Frances Finnegan 2004 *Do Penance or Perish: Magdalen Asylums in Ireland.* Oxford University Press, Oxford.

legal advisor, Colm MacGeehin, whose long battle for survivors reminds one of why the oft-maligned legal profession exists: the pursuit of justice. To Sheila Martin, whose detailed and painstaking research first alerted me to some of the more shocking aspects of the surgery in the Lourdes Hospital, my thanks. Without the support of Stewart O'Connell of Johnswood Press, who printed at cost, gifted the design and layout, and secured generous offers from suppliers, Tony Swan of Swan Paper and Pamela Monaghan of Print Finishers who donated paper and binding, this report might not have seen the light of day. The same observation could be made in respect of SoS National Executive members, particularly Marie and Billy Crean, whose unswerving support could always be relied upon. Finally, I wish to acknowledge the inestimable contribution made by Kathleen Naughten and Olivia Kearney, an unfailing source of detailed information on SoS, especially its early years.

SoS's road towards justice has been long and arduous. I hope that this report will be a milestone on that journey towards truth and justice, and that the testimony of survivors here in Ireland may ultimately help to stem the mainstreaming of these destructive operations in resource poor countries by misguided European doctors.

Marie O'Connor
Dublin
June 2011

# Executive Summary

Symphysiotomy is a childbirth operation that severs one of the main pelvic joints, sundering the pubic bones and unhinging the pelvis. A related operation, pubiotomy, which splits the pubic bone rather than the symphysis joint and results in a 'compound fracture of the pelvis',[7] was also performed. At least 1,500 of these operations were recorded here from 1944-92: most were carried out in 'voluntary' or private hospitals under the control of the Catholic dioceses of Dublin, Armagh, and Cork and Ross. Around 180 symphysiotomy mothers are believed to survive in Ireland today.

The surgery was revived in Ireland as an elective or non-emergency procedure to deal with pelvic disproportion, lack of fit between the baby's head and its mother's pelvis, a 'complication' later found to be non-existent.[8] Symphysiotomy and pubiotomy were carried out under almost unprecedented circumstances, during late pregnancy, and, even more aberrantly, following the birth of a baby born by Caesarean section.

These operations were shrouded in considerable secrecy. Patient consent was generally not sought, nor were women necessarily informed of their surgery after the event, even by their general practitioners. Several decades elapsed before many understood that their pelvises had been broken.

Although some wore binders in hospital, symphysiotomy mothers were generally nursed in the same way as women who did not have surgery. They were discharged home unable to walk, usually after ten or twelve days, without binders, advice or painkillers. This failure of care continued in the community and led in many cases to catastrophic consequences. Walking disabilities, chronic pain and lifelong incontinence are common. Babies born by symphysiotomy were

---

[7]  Richard E Tottenham 1931 *A Handbook of Midwifery.* Churchill, London, 242.
[8]  Kieran O Driscoll, Declan Meagher with Peter Boylan 1993 *Active Management of Labor The Dublin Experience.* 3rd ed. Mosby, London, 65.

generally placed in intensive care for 10 or 12 days, or more. One was brain damaged. Others died: hospital reports indicate that one baby in ten did not survive the operation.

Many of the health and disability benefits promised to women by the government in 2003 have been reduced or, in some cases, discontinued, while some were never provided. Contrary to official claims, no comprehensive package is in place today to meet survivors' health care needs. Access to services is, and has been, a postcode lottery. Women's inability to pursue a recalcitrant bureaucracy has led to double, or even treble, discrimination, with age combining with disability and geography to ensure that those most in need are often least looked after.

While the authorities have been under pressure to mount an independent inquiry for a decade, little progress has been made. An external review promised by government in 2003 was later withdrawn. A television exposé in 2010 led to a ministerial request for an internal report from a private body closely associated with these operations, the Institute of Obstetricians and Gynaecologists. This was to have been completed in April 2010, but no report has issued. One report that may have been commissioned by the Institute may have been withdrawn, and a second one has now been commissioned by the Department of Health.

The Institute's position, which has been adopted by the authorities, is that symphysiotomy was the norm for difficult births until it was 'replaced' by Caesarean section in the 1950s. Another, somewhat contradictory, account advanced by several leading obstetricians has it that Caesarean section was the standard operation for obstructed labour, and that symphysiotomy was carried out to avoid the medical risks associated with repeat Caesarean. Both of these narratives agree, however, that symphysiotomy was done for medical reasons and that it was safe for mothers. These are myths.

Symphysiotomy never succeeded in establishing itself as a norm for obstructed labour. Contemporaneous accounts show that the surgery was dogged by controversy even in 1777, and was widely shunned by doctors, then and later, on account of its dangers. Pubiotomy, a later variant, came to be regarded with even greater suspicion. By the mid-1940s, when symphysiotomy and pubiotomy were revived at the National Maternity Hospital (NMH) Dublin, these operations were not considered acceptable medical practice in the English-speaking world. By 1944, Caesarean section was well established in Ireland as the norm for difficult births. Ireland was the sole country in the Western world to practice symphysiotomy and pubiotomy in the mid to late 20$^{th}$ century.

Symphysiotomy has been represented as a solution to the problems posed by repeat Caesareans in an era when family limitation was unknown. Demographics show, however, that family size in Ireland was shrinking even before the 1940s and this trend intensified in later decades, particularly from the 1960s. Hospital records for these decades show that these operations continued to be practiced in Cork hospitals until the late 1970s and in Drogheda until the early 1980s, and later instances have also been reported by survivors.

While Caesarean section was the norm for obstructed labour by 1944, it was (and remains) an operation that, once performed, tended to be repeated. Good practice was generally seen to limit the number of Caesareans that could safely be performed, however: three was the upper limit as the Lourdes Hospital, for example. Caesarean section was therefore seen by doctors as limiting family size.

Religious beliefs appeared to be central to the latter day practice of these operations in Ireland. Prominent practitioners of symphysiotomy were at the centre of an informal network that included Archbishop John Charles McQuaid, and several were members of Catholic Action groups, such as the Knights of Columbanus and the Guild of Saints Luke, Cosmas and Damian, a medical association dedicated to putting Catholic teaching into clinical practice. The writings of leading symphysiotomy revivalists at NMH, such as Dr Alex Spain and Dr Arthur Barry, are indicative of moral, not medical, difficulties with Caesarean. While they accepted its safety, they saw it as morally hazardous. Caesarean section was seen by them as the gateway to 'the mutilating operation of sterilisation'[9] and other practices, such as 'the improper prevention of pregnancy'[10] Symphysiotomy was intended to offer 'a permanent cure for disproportion' — an alternative to Caesarean section in selected cases — and a lifetime of unrestricted childbearing. Personal belief systems took precedence over patient safety.

Survivors' testimony, borne out by historical and medical writings, suggests that, in teaching hospitals, such as the National Maternity and the Lourdes Hospitals, the surgery was also driven by the need to train medical students. Symphysiotomy, an operation so simple that it did not even require electricity, was seen in the 1940s as an invaluable substitute for Caesarean section in Africa, for example, where the Medical Missionaries of Mary had a growing number of clinics and hospitals. The surgery has been extensively reported there from 1950-99, and Holles St Hospital is credited with its export.

The 'symphysiotomy experiment'[11] at NMH lasted until the mid-1960s. It continued at the Lourdes Hospital, however, until the mid-1980s. Symphysiotomy was performed there under extreme circumstances, before labour began and after a baby was born. Described in detail in hospital reports, these cases constituted a significant body of data that may well have been useful in clinics overseas. One hospital owned by the Medical Missionaries of Mary in Nigeria, in Afikpo, Ebonyi State, has published data on over 1,000 symphysiotomies.[12] Symphysiotomy is now being promoted in resource poor countries as a 'safe', low cost alternative to Caesarean section.

---

9    Alex Spain 1949 'Apologia for Symphysiotomy and Pubiotomy'. *Journal of Obstetrics and Gynaecology of the British Empire* 56 Aug: 577.

10   Arthur Barry 1954 'Conservatism in Obstetrics'. *Transactions of the 6th International Congress of Catholic Doctors* John Fleetwood Ed. Guild of St Luke, SS Cosmas and Damian, Dublin, 122. In Jacqueline K Morrisey 2004 *An examination of the relationship between the Catholic Church and the medical profession in Ireland in the period 1922 – 1992, with particular emphasis on the impact of this relationship in the field of reproductive medicine.* . Unpublished PhD thesis University College Dublin, 155.

11   Ibid, 157.

12   IM Sunday-Adeoye, P Okonta and D Twomey 2004 'Symphysiotomy at the Mater Misericordiae Hospital Afikpo, Ebonyi State of Nigeria (1982-1999): a review of 1013 cases'. *Journal of Obstetrics and Gynaecology* Jan 24 (5): 525-529.

Done in Ireland at a time when Caesarean section offered a much safer alternative, these dangerous operations constituted medical negligence; performed without patient consent, they were illegal, and constituted battery. They breached constitutional rights, such as the right to bodily integrity, the right to privacy, including self-determination, and the right to refuse medical care or treatment. They also violated human rights. Obliging a mother to endure prolonged labour before sundering her pelvis under local anaesthetic, and requiring her to give birth despite the pain of a severed symphysis amounted to cruel and inhuman treatment in the absence of medical necessity.

These operations, carried out, as they were, by male doctors exercising control over women's reproductive lives, reflected the strength of a patriarchal culture marked by paternalism and clericalism, where the power of the medical profession intertwined with that of the Catholic Church. The practice of symphysiotomy was a product of a consultant-controlled and highly interventionist hospital culture that reduced midwives to medical underlings. Marked by a collegial, if collusive, loyalty that was apparently underpinned by fear, this culture ignored the patient's right to decline surgery and led to a professional silence that endangered patients.

Regulatory failure in Ireland allowed the widespread practice of these aberrant operations for four decades. Hospital clinical reports detailing these operations were sent to medical bodies with responsibility for professional standards in the area, such as the Royal College of Obstetricians and Gynaecologists in London and the Institute of Obstetricians and Gynaecologists in Dublin. State regulators, such as the Department of Health, the regional health boards and the Medical Council, also turned a blind eye.

'Bodily Harm' concludes that the latter day practice of symphysiotomy was a form of institutional abuse for which no person or agency has ever been held to account. Truth and justice for survivors demand equitable access to comprehensive benefits and entitlements, an independent inquiry into the surgery, and the setting aside of the statute of limitations, which has acted as a barrier to redress.

# I 'A daily crucifixion': the unhinging of the pelvis

*'Every time I look at a crucifix, it reminds me of me.
It's been a daily crucifixion.'*

> Máire O'Sullivan, an 85-year-old survivor of
> symphysiotomy in Wicklow.

## First babies, younger mothers

Symphysiotomy is a birth operation that severs one of the principal pelvic joints, the symphysis pubis, sundering the pubic bones and unhinging the pelvis. A simple, if destructive, procedure, symphysiotomy was widely practiced in Ireland from 1944-84, with over 1,500 of these operations reportedly being carried out. One instance has been reported as late as 1992. Some mothers appear to have been subjected to a related operation, pubiotomy, that cuts the pubic bone close to the symphysis pubis, and results in a compound fracture of the pelvis.[13]

Many of these women were having their first baby. There was also a trend towards younger mothers: symphysiotomy was seen as particularly suitable for young women having their first baby.[14] Many of those operated upon at the Lourdes Hospital in the early 1960s, for example, were in their mid to late 20s.

These 'new' procedures were almost invariably performed by senior doctors of consultant rank, with some being done by professors of obstetrics and gynaecology. Many were carried out by the masters of two of the main Dublin maternity hospitals.

---

[13] Richard E Tottenham 1931 *A Handbook of Midwifery.* Churchill, London, 242.
[14] Jacqueline K Morrisey 2004 *An examination of the relationship between the Catholic Church and the medical profession in Ireland in the period 1922 – 1992, with particular emphasis on the impact of this relationship in the field of reproductive medicine.* Unpublished PhD thesis University College Dublin, 188.

While around 180 symphysiotomy mothers are believed to survive today, the   exact number is not known. Women who had two operations under general anaesthetic for the birth of the same baby may not know they were symphysiotomised. In many cases, hospital staff apparently neglected to inform women that they had undergone surgery. No hospital in Ireland has written collectively to its former patients to inform them of their operations. Indeed, one epicentre of symphysiotomy in Dublin, the National Maternity Hospital (NMH) may not be in a position to do so, as it has destroyed its medical records from the 1950s and 60s.

---

**1. Myths and red herrings**
'From about 1920 until 1960, the operations of symphsyiotomy were employed in selected cases in Dublin, mainly in the National Maternity Hospital and the Coombe Hospital.' John Bonnar, Chairman of the Institute of Obstetricians and Gynaecologists, 2001.[15]

---

**Persistent and widespread**
Contrary to what the Institute of Obstetricians and Gynaecologists (IOG) has indicated,  symphysiotomy did not cease in Ireland in 1960, nor was it confined to Dublin, particularly. The surgery persisted at Our Lady of  Lourdes Hospital until 1984: doctors there probably did more of these operations, proportionately, than their Dublin colleagues. Of the 1 500 recorded symphysiotomies in Ireland, over 800 were done in three so-called voluntary hospitals, the National Maternity and the Coombe in Dublin, and the Lourdes in Drogheda. NMH reports show that 272 symphysiotomies were carried out there from 1944-66[16]. The Coombe Lying-in Hospital (as it was then known) was another centre:

---

[15]  John Bonnar 2001 Letter to Dr Jim Kiely, Chief Medical Officer, Department of Health and Children. 4 May.

[16]  *National Maternity Hospital Report 1948 Irish Journal of Medical Science 1949. National Maternity Hospital Report 1955 Irish Journal of Medical Science 1956. Royal Academy of Medicine Transactions 1958 Irish Journal of Medical Science* 1958:542. In Jacqueline K Morrisey 2004 op cit, 158, 173-4.

pelvic division was as common there as it was at NMH.[17] Coombe Hospital reports show that 147 symphysiotomies were carried out there from 1950-63[18]. The number of surgeries carried out at the Lourdes Hospital is disputed, however. Minister of State Brian Lenihan TD told the Dáil on 27 May 2003 that his Department (Health) had been informed by the North-Eastern Health Board that 188 of these operations had been performed at the Lourdes from 1955-82.[19] Six weeks later, however, that figure almost doubled: on 7 July 2003, the same Board informed Jan O'Sullivan TD that 334 symphysiotomies had been done at the Lourdes over an unspecified time period.[20] Sheila Martin's research indicates, however, that the total number is around 400 for the period 1956-1984.[21] Records for earlier years are incomplete.

The surgery was more persistent and widespread than has been hitherto reported. Thanks to the teaching role of NMH, the Coombe[22] and the Lourdes, the surgery spread far and wide. While the bulk of the operations appear to have been performed in private or voluntary Catholic hospitals, the surgery was also carried out in public or state hospitals and some were done in private maternity or nursing homes. It persisted at the Lourdes Hospital, until 1984. The Southern Health Board reported that 26 had been done at Sr Finbarr's Hospital, Cork, from 1941-82; and 25 in the Erinville, from '1954-'mid-1970s'.[23] The surgery has been reported by survivors as late as 1992 at Dublin's NMH; 1978 at Cork's Erinville Hospital; 1977 at Waterford's Airmount Hospital (then run by the Medical Missionaries of Mary[24]); and 1974 at Dublin's Rotunda Hospital.

Other hospitals that performed symphysiotomies in the 1960s include St James's, Dublin, the Bons Secours, Cork, Dundalk Hospital and the

---

[17] Ibid, 175.
[18] Coombe Lying-In Hospital Reports 1950-63 *Irish Journal of Medical Science* 1951-64.
[19] Brian Lenihan TD 2003 Dáil Debates. 'Hospital Practices.' Vol 567 No 5 Col 1008-9 27 May.
[20] Tadhg O'Brien 2003 Letter to Jan O'Sullivan TD. 7 July.
[21] Sheila Martin 2009 *Symphysiotomy at Our Lady of Lourdes*. Unpublished diploma thesis, 1.
[22] Jacqueline K Morrisey 2004 op cit, 182.
[23] Sean Hurley 2003. Letter to Jan O'Sullivan TD. 11 July.
[24] http://www.waterfordcity.ie/departments/archives/pages/maternity.htm

Coombe Hospital, where one was reported as late as 1969. Three cases were reported by the Western Health Board at Portiuncula Hospital, Ballinasloe, Co Galway,[25] (which was owned by the Franciscan Missionaries of the Divine Motherhood until 2001). Other hospitals where the operation has been reported by survivors include University College Hospital, Galway (where the hospital was 'unable', without additional resources, to provide the information sought by Jan O'Sullivan TD[26]); Limerick Regional Hospital (where, according to the Mid-Western Health Board, 'no records' of this procedure' existed[27]); Port Laoise Hospital (where, according to the Midland Health Board, no symphysiotomies were carried out[28]), and a Dublin nursing home, Stella Maris (which had a close relationship with NMH).

---

### 2. Myths and red herrings
'Many of these cases [at NMH and the Coombe in the 1940s and '50s] were emergency admissions with obstructed labour.' John Bonnar, Chairman of the Institute of Obstetricians and Gynaecologists, 2001.[29]

---

### A planned procedure
This assertion is groundless. National Maternity and Coombe Hospital reports bear out the fact that symphysiotomy was performed as an elective, or non-emergency, procedure. While symphysiotomy was generally regarded as an operation of last resort in the English-speaking world — to be performed only when all else had failed — the same tolerance was not extended to pubiotomy. Both were revived at NMH as 'a cure for disproportion' (lack of fit between the baby's head and the mother's pelvis), one that was intended in many cases to replace Caesarean section.[30]

---

[25]  Chris Kane 2003. Letter to Jan O'Sullivan TD. 15 July.
[26]  Ibid.
[27]  John O'Brien 2003. Letter to Jan O'Sullivan TD. 14 July.
[28]  Joe Martin 2003. Letter to Jan O'Sullivan TD. 30 June.
[29]  John Bonnar 2001 op cit.
[30]  Jacqueline K Morrisey 2004 op cit, 154.

Many patients had a pelvic x-ray during pregnancy (a common procedure in earlier decades), suggesting that disproportion was often diagnosed before a woman went into labour. Most of these operations were carried out during labour, but some were done under other circumstances. Dr Alex Spain, who revived symphysiotomy at Holles St, advocated that, in certain cases, the pelvis should be cut before labour began.[31] Matilda Behan (her real name) was admitted to NMH in May 1958, ten days before her third baby was due. Four days later, she was brought to theatre: 'I wasn't in labour but I thought it was for my [Caesarean] section. The next thing, I was physically restrained. I had a local anaesthetic, and was fully awake and they had this circular saw. I was screaming, asking what they were doing. They said "new procedure". They told me they broke the pelvis bone and my hips were dislocated. The baby was still inside me'.[32] The 'circular saw' is likely to have been a type of chain saw known as a 'Gigli' saw, which that was widely used to cut the pubic bone in pubiotomy.

These operations were also carried out at NMH in a small number of cases following the birth of a baby by Caesarean section.[33]

Women diagnosed with a minor degree of disproportion who were having their first baby at NMH were permitted a 'trial of labour' — a chance to see if they could birth their baby themselves — before a decision was taken to proceed with surgery.[34] Where no such trial of labour was permitted, women were often still required to spend a great many hours in labour before the procedure was performed.

Pubiotomy was also performed. In this operation (also confusingly referred to as 'symphysiotomy'), the pubic bone was cut to the left of the *symphysis pubis* joint. The rule at NMH was that pubiotomy was to be carried out in the event that the joint of the *symphysis* could not be

---

[31] 'Royal Academy of Medicine Transactions 1950' *Irish Journal of Medical Science* 1950: 861 In ibid, 162.
[32] Aine O'Connor 2002 'When giving birth becomes a mother's worst nightmare'. *Sunday Independent* 5 May.
[33] Jacqueline K Morrisey 2004 op cit, 173.
[34] Ibid, 158.

located.[35] However, Matilda Behan's testimony indicates that the operation may have been carried out more widely than this policy would suggest.

**Symphysiotomy during pregnancy**
Three types of symphysiotomy were recorded in detail at Our Lady of Lourdes Hospital, Drogheda, all of them planned or non-emergency. The first was formally classified as 'elective', that is, performed before a mother went into labour. Some women admitted on their due date had a symphysiotomy; others were symphysiotomised some weeks or days before their due date. All of these operations were done under general anaesthetic. One mother aged 25 was seven and a half months' pregnant when her pelvis was severed: she was sent home, hobbling, to await the birth of her first child. Today, 47 years on, she still suffers from the side effects of the surgery and has had three operations on her back, all, she believes, stemming from her symphysiotomy. Her last surgery was in November 2009, when bone was removed from her spinal chord and a metal plate inserted.

Symphysiotomy could not always be relied upon to ensure a vaginal birth, however. In these cases, mothers who had been symphysiotomised went on to have a Caesarean section, under general anaesthetic, for the birth of the same baby. One mother who was having her third child in 1962-63 had her pelvis cut before labour began, the operation failed and the baby was finally delivered by Caesarean section three weeks after her symphysiotomy following a seven hour labour.[36]

Women continued to be routinely symphysiotomised at the Lourdes during pregnancy until the late 1960s.[37]

---

[35] Ibid, 178.
[36] *Our Lady of Lourdes Hospital Drogheda International Missionary Training Centre Clinical Report* Maternity Department 1962-63: 35.
[37] *Our Lady of Lourdes Hospital Drogheda International Missionary Training Centre Clinical Report* Maternity Department 1970-71: 43.

**During labour**

The second type of symphysiotomy was performed on women whose labour had already begun. Despite the widespread use of pelvic x-rays at the Lourdes, there seems to have been a practice at the unit of allowing some women seen as 'candidates' for symphysiotomy to go over their due date. Eleven of the 48 women symphysiotomised at the Lourdes in 1960-'61, for example, were overdue: the babies ranged in weight from 6lbs 5oz to 11lbs 15oz.[38] The failure to induce a mother suspected of disproportion during pregnancy was curious. Vera Kennedy recalled how 'they discovered the baby was breech at eight months. She was too big. They did 2 x-rays to see if my pelvis was big enough. But they let me go over [my due date] 18 days. …. They knew she was big, that she was breech, they could have done a Caesarean.' A breech presentation appeared to be an indication for symphysiotomy at the Lourdes, as was, extraordinarily, a brow presentation, and a face, and babies presenting in these positions were delivered in this way at the unit until 1974-'75.[39]

Two symphysiotomy techniques were employed at the Lourdes during labour. One was the so-called open method, which entailed an incision in the abdomen 'large enough for the operator to see'[40] and was carried out on mothers in early labour. The other method, a partial, subcutaneous incision described as 'Zarate's', was much more common, however. For example, of the 48 cases recorded at the Lourdes Hospital in 1960-61, Zarate's was the method employed in 40 of them.[41] Performed on women whose labour was more advanced, Zarate's method, while being less invasive, was seen by symphysiotomy practitioners in Africa as high risk.[42]

---

[38] *Our Lady of Lourdes Hospital Drogheda International Missionary Training Centre Clinical Report* Maternity Department 1960-'61: 35-9.

[39] *Our Lady of Lourdes Hospital Drogheda International Missionary Training Centre Clinical Report* Maternity Department 1972-'73: 53.

[40] Sheila Martin 2009 op cit, 7.

[41] *Our Lady of Lourdes Hospital Drogheda International Missionary Training Centre Clinical Report* Maternity Department 1960-61; 40.

[42] D Crichton and EK Seedat 1963 'The technique of symphysiotomy'. *South African Medical Journal* 37: 227-31.

Mothers selected for symphysiotomy during labour were frequently left by hospital staff to languish for hours or even days in labour. The policy of giving all first time mothers — x-rayed and deemed in need of 'a little more room'[43] — a trial of labour led to long labours. This policy seems to have been extended to all women at the Lourdes.[44] Whether or not mothers were given an opportunity to give birth themselves, medical opinion generally held that a cervical dilatation of five cms[45] was required before a symphysiotomy could be carried out. Babies occasionally died while hospital staff waited for labour to 'progress'. At the Lourdes Hospital, where symphysiotomy could be carried out at any time from 27 weeks' gestation onwards, most pelvis cutting procedures were performed during labour, at four cms' dilatation.[46] Pre-symphysiotomy labours ranged from 6-48 hours in 1958-9. One woman was left in labour for 44 hours in 1960-61, a hospital report noted.[47] These long labours — arduous even by the standards of the time — culminated in symphysiotomy.

Survivors have described how, without warning, a consultant would appear in the delivery unit, and give orders to prepare them for surgery. These labour ward operations were reportedly witnessed by large numbers of staff, and were performed upon women whose feet were manacled in stirrups or held in the 'stranded beetle' [lithotomy] position that the surgery required. One mother described the experience: 'He [Dr Gerard Connolly] came in with a big entourage. It was very invasive, you were tied up [in stirrups], you had no control. There was a good crowd there, nurses, other people behind him, two or three other doctors, I took them to be, juniors, students.'

---

[43] Jacqueline K Morrisey 2004 op cit, 158.

[44] Gerard Connolly 1966 *Royal Academy of Medicine in Ireland Transactions: Section of Obstetrics The annual reports of the Rotunda, Coombe and National Maternity Hospitals for the year 1964*. 7 Jan.

[45] Crichton D and Seedat EK 1962. Symphysiotomy: technique, indications and limitations. *The Lancet* (i): 554-59.

[46] Sheila Martin 2009 op cit, 5.

[47] *Our Lady of Lourdes Hospital Drogheda International Missionary Training Centre Clinical Report* Maternity Department 1960-61: 36.

A decision was taken at Holles St in 1952 that symphysiotomy and, presumably, pubiotomy would henceforth be carried out under local anaesthetic, as a general anaesthetic was deemed too risky to the fetus.[48] This also seems to have been the policy at the Lourdes for the Zarate type of symphysiotomy performed during labour. While local anaesthetic was safer for the mother as well as the baby, its use meant that the birth was extremely painful, even when the anaesthetic was supplemented with pain relief in the form of gas and air. Teresa Moroney likened the experience to 'getting teeth pulled ... They did it under a local anaesthetic, but I noted the feeling, the sensations'. Women were required to give birth after the operation, notwithstanding the post-operative pain of an unhinged pelvis. Mothers whose babies did not come faced further hours of labour, 14 hours in one case.[49]

Episiotomy, a surgical incision widening the opening of the birth canal, was frequently performed to expedite the birth. The capacity of the operation to enable normal birth was open to question. While some mothers within this group of survivors succeeded in giving birth without medical assistance, many had a forceps or a vacuum delivery, where the baby is extracted through force of suction by means of a cap fitted to its head and attached to a vacuum machine. And if the symphysiotomy failed, as it not infrequently did, the baby was delivered by Caesarean section. Ann Moloney describes how she was left in labour for two days following her symphysiotomy before doctors finally performed a Caesarean section. Such manifold failures were also described in NMII reports. Arthur Barry related how 'on two occasions, owing to difficulty in finding the [symphysis] joint, it was found necessary to cut the [pubic] bone. On one occasion, as a result of persistent [uterine] inertia, [Caesarean] section eventually proved necessary'.[50] Such birth experiences must have been harrowing for the women concerned.

---

[48] Jacqueline K Morrisey 2004 op cit, 171-2.
[49] *Our Lady of Lourdes Hospital Drogheda International Missionary Training Centre Clinical Report* Maternity Department 1960-61:35.
[50] Arthur Barry 1951 *National Maternity Hospital Report 1951:* 7-8. In Jacqueline K Morrisey 2004 op cit, 171-2.

**Following Caesarean section**

The third category of symphysiotomy at the Lourdes Hospital was done in the aftermath of Caesarean section. These 'on the way out' symphysiotomies, as they were termed, were without precedent[51] and the grounds for these procedures remain uncertain. They were usually performed after a baby had been delivered by Caesarean section under general anaesthetic, while the abdomen was being closed. Until the 1970s, a classic Caesarean section generally entailed vertical cuts into the abdomen and uterus. Vertical cuts were preferred by some consultant obstetricians at the Lourdes for Caesarean section: these incisions, which left women with long, disfiguring scars down their abdomen, persisted there long after they had been discontinued in other hospitals.[52] Seven Caesarean symphysiotomies were performed in Drogheda in 1966-7 on women ranging in age from 22 to 30.[53] One 18 year-old mother was subjected to the double procedure in 1969. It was her first and only pregnancy. Some of these 'on the way out' symphysiotomies failed: these mothers went on to have a Caesarean section in a future birth. Caesarean symphysiotomies continued to be common at the Lourdes until 1970, when it was discontinued.[54]

**Consent**

Whatever type of symphysiotomy was performed, survivors have reported that doctors did not seek their consent prior to operating upon them, nor did they give them any information about the nature of the operation, its likely consequences, its known risks, or the existence of a safer alternative: Caesarean section. Not one mother reported that her consent had been sought prior to surgery.

---

[51] Kenneth Bjorklund 2002 'Minimally invasive surgery for obstructed labour: a review of symphysiotomy during the twentieth century (including 5000 cases)'. *British Journal of Obstetrics and Gynaecology* 109 (3): 236-48.

[52] Maureen Harding Clark 2006 *The Lourdes Hospital Inquiry An Inquiry into peripartum hysterectomy at Our Lady of Lourdes Hospital Drogheda Report of Judge Maureen Harding Clark SC.* Stationary Office, Dublin, 226, 230.

[53] *Our Lady of Lourdes Hospital Drogheda International Missionary Training Centre Clinical Report* Maternity Department 1966-67; 43-7.

[54] *Our Lady of Lourdes Hospital Drogheda International Missionary Training Centre Clinical Report* Maternity Department 1970-71: 43.

**Post surgery care**
The same failure to give information was evident after the operation. Although many mothers were wide awake while the surgery was being performed, they had little or no understanding of what was being done and hospital staff reportedly neglected to explain after the event. Sarah Long says she was told by staff that she had had a Caesarean section, but such disinformation was uncommon, it seems. However, only a very small minority of women reported leaving hospital with the knowledge that their pelvis had been cut and several decades elapsed before many understood the nature of their surgery.

Mothers invariably describe the post-operative pain in the strongest possible terms. Those who had had surgery wide awake were generally sedated after giving birth for a day or so: Largactil was the drug of choice at the Lourdes.[55]

Symphysiotomy patients report being nursed in the same way as women who had not been operated upon. Their fellow patients had to lift their legs in and out of bed for them, because survivors could not move them of their own volition. Instead of immoblising a mother with a broken pelvis, she was usually forced to walk, albeit in agony. Some women were permitted to remain in bed for several days, while others were required to get up almost immediately, depending on the thinking that was in vogue at the time. One woman recalled how she was 'whipped out the next morning. Two nurses ... got me straight out of bed... It's all changed, you're out straightaway after an operation now, that's what she [the sister] said'. Another mother was required to walk by a hospital physiotherapist: 'she told me to get out of bed ... The pain was excruciating'.

The failure on the part of hospital staff to care for these surgical patients was striking. While 'tight wiring' of the pelvis was essential to minimise disability,[56] a significant number of women were left without binders. Nuala Kavanagh related what happened to a pelvis that had been left

---

55  Sheila Martin 2009 op cit, 9.
56  Seamus O'Friel 2004 Letter *Irish Times* 22 July.

unbound: 'Bone grew in the space. It's like an abcess on my right side…It didn't knit where it was supposed to knit.' Historically, in cases where the symphysis ruptured naturally during childbirth, strict bed rest was prescribed in conjunction with the wearing of a pelvic binder.[57] In these cases, where the pelvis had been ruptured surgically, no such treatment was prescribed, apparently.

Mothers were generally separated from their babies after birth, unaware initially that their children were in intensive care. One described how hospital midwives gave her no information: 'I didn't realise he was in an incubator, that he was in intensive care. They brought him to me on day five [after the birth]. I wasn't able to hold him, I wasn't able to feed him.' Another woman underlined the pain of this enforced separation: 'it was very hard on a mother, when you were yearning for your baby.'

Irish hospital data indicate that one baby in ten did not survive the operation.[58] Prolonged labour could be hard on a baby starved of oxygen in a womb left to contract too hard for too long.

Babies who survived the surgery — at risk of brain damage and other internal injuries — were generally placed in intensive care for ten or twelve days. One mother described her daughter's condition: 'she was so sore she would cry when they moved the incubator. She had a cerebral swelling. Her face and her head were distorted.'

**Care in the community**
The postnatal period — a time of unique vulnerability for all women — was infinitely more difficult for a mother with a broken pelvis. Lack of aftercare appears to have been the norm, however. Many women were discharged from hospital ten or twelve days after the birth, without medical advice or painkillers. One commented: 'they should

---

[57] Zhiyong Hou et al 2011 'Severe postpartum disruption of the pelvic ring: report of two cases and review of the literature.' *Patient Safety in Surgery* 5:2. 3 January. http://www.pssjournal.com/content/5/1/2
[58] Kevin Feeney 1956 *Coombe Lying-In Hospital Report 1956 Irish Journal of Medical Science* 1957. In Jacqueline K Morrisey 2004 op cit, 190.

have advised us on what to do and what not to do. They should have advised our husbands ... There was no special care. They never followed any woman up.'

For most, the after effects of the surgery were devastating. Women reported being unable to get out of bed, unable to walk, unable to sleep. They were unable to look after their newborns, unable to mind their other children, unable to care for themselves. Yet there was no hospital follow up in the community, it seems, nor any community care. Some women complained of lack of support from general practitioners, who generally saw their patients six weeks after the birth for a postnatal examination. Public health nurses visits at this time were hardly mentioned: they did not appear to play a salient role in women's postnatal care.

Deprived of medical care in the community, women tended to turn to their mothers for general nursing and baby care. Siblings and other family members often helped in cases where there were other children to be minded. Like others, Vera Kennedy spent two months in her mother's house. She described herself as 'walking' when she was discharged from hospital, 'hobbling, you'd call it... I don't know how I managed...I was in agony.' Nuala Kavanagh, whose baby had been extremely difficult to birth and whose pelvis had been left unbound, also underlines the pain: 'I was crying with the pain. It was as if my leg fell apart. ...It was a nightmare, like coming out of a crash.' She was nursed by her mother: 'I used to have my leg propped up: my mother would tie a bolster [case] around me at night and pin it. .. She was always packing my back with cushions and pillows to relieve the pain.'

In addition to being denied appropriate care, symphysiotomy mothers were also deprived of the simple pleasures of motherhood. The joy of taking a new baby out for a walk, for example, to be admired by friends and neighbours, or making a social call. And bonding could be difficult with a child whose birth was traumatic.

### 3. Myths and red herrings

'The joint heals with laying down of dense connective [scar] tissue ... Reported long term problems include walking difficulties, pelvic joint pain and urinary incontinence. These may subside after 3 to 6 months: The Institute of Obstetricians and Gynaecologists, 2010.[59]

### Long term complications

Women also reported other health problems at this time, in addition to pain, disability and continence issues. Wound infections at the site of the operation were not uncommon. Peg Prendergast was particularly unfortunate: she suffered a ruptured bladder and was kept in hospital for six months following her childbirth surgery.

Breda Lynch says it took 'the best part of seven years to get back to half normal: Her case was not an isolated one. In Nuala Kavanagh's case, the pain persisted for eight years, then 'subsided somewhat. I got so many infections down there; I got urinary infections as well. Those infections went on for eight years: Serious, long term complications have been widely reported. Like many another survivor, Sarah Long, 77, describes her gait as 'waddling; She has difficulty lying on her sides and suffers from chronic pain in all her bones, particularly in her back and legs. Incontinence is an issue and she also has a prolapsed uterus. She underlines the psychological effects of the surgery: 'mental scarring forever...chronic depression... severe panic attacks, phobias about hospitals, surgeons, nurses and doctors, anger management issues, diminished confidence: Sarah's health profile is fairly typical of survivors of symphysiotomy.

The operation often left mothers disabled, in pain, incontinent, and, in some cases, their marital and other family relationships stressed. Rosemary Harte sums up the experience of many when she says: 'the pain, the backache, the incontinence, never went away'. In some cases,

---

[59]  Institute of Obstetricians and Gynaecologists 2010 'Statement on symphysiotomy:
17 Feb.

the breaking of the pelvis led to consequences that took a few years to manifest: one mother, who had the surgery on her first child, said her pelvis 'shot out' when she was having her third baby. One mother reported that her pelvic bone had broken, and she attributed this to her symphysiotomy, done 41 years previously. Some mothers have had repeated surgery. Josephine Lawlor, for example, has had surgery on her neck and back, while Miriam O'Keefe has had 'at least five' operations to repair her bladder. One of her specialists told her there was no support given to the pelvis after her symphysiotomy: 'my spine has twisted from rocking loosely into my pelvis'. Many women have chronic bladder problems, either as a direct result of their surgery or as a consequence of an unstable pelvis, or both. Some, additionally, suffer from bowel difficulties.

For almost every woman, symphysiotomy led to at least some degree of permanent disability. Most experience marked difficulty in ascending or descending a staircase. Some women reported severe walking difficulties persisting for a year or more that, while they improved over time, never resolved. Those most damaged by the surgery suffer from pelvic instability. One woman described how difficult it was to walk with an unstable pelvis: 'I needed a lot of intermittences of rest ... The pelvis clicks, I can hear it ... There's a huge gap there, you can see it on the x-ray'.

Symphysiotomy mothers today range in age from their late 50s to their late 80s, spanning nearly two generations. Age has sharpened their pain and exacerbated their injuries. One mother who has been attending SoS meetings for a decade says many survivors are now in wheelchairs, or have walking aids. In her own case, she says there has been a definite disimprovement over the past 20 years: 'as you get older, the pains get worse, in the legs, in the feet...even my toes, the pain would wake me at night'. The effects on the body of an unstable pelvis over 30 or 40 years are wide ranging: another mother says her feet have become flat due to the waddling caused by symphysiotomy. Mary Maguire reports that she is half an inch short in her right leg. Dolores Dooley now suffers from a prolapsed bladder.

Chronic pain is an extremely common side-effect. Marred by disability and moulded by pain, some suffer in their backs, their legs, their feet, their toes. Some survivors report pain in the groin, and in some cases, this pain has spread to the base of the neck and the upper arms. For some women, the quest for effective pain relief has been lifelong. Some believe in hot showers and evening primrose oil, while others prefer to take medication. The long term use of painkillers appears to be common. A small number of women have attended a specialist clinic for pain relieving injections. Others take anti-inflammatory drugs in injection or tablet form, while still others wear morphine patches. These medications are supplemented in some cases by over the counter preparations. Some wear a pelvic binder daily, and bed rest continues to be a necessity for a number. Many have tried a range of conventional and alternative health practitioners. Some have consulted faith healers and joined prayer groups, while others have found physiotherapy helpful, and still others find relief from complementary therapies, such as reflexology or acupuncture.

**A lifetime of loss**
The consequences of the surgery were complex and multi layered. Symphysiotomy did not just affect individual women, it impacted on couples. Its side effects were psychological as well as physical. Some of these side effects rarely, if ever, featured in the medical literature on symphysiotomy. Genital injuries made sexual relations extremely difficult, if not impossible: marriages occasionally buckled under the strain. Dolores Dooley recounts how she was only married 12 months when she was symphysiotomised: 'my childhood sweetheart husband got back an invalid and a totally different-thinking wife'. For some, sexual relations belonged to a former life, a life prior to surgery. One mother consulted her general practitioner: 'I had to go to the doctor, it was a few years after. The doctor didn't tell me what was wrong with me, no one did. He didn't examine me, no one did'. The operation was followed by sterility in several cases, at least. Marjorie McDonogh explained: 'I had no more children after the symphysiotomy on purpose, because of fear of childbirth'.

Symphysiotomy could also be seen to affect families. Children were deeply affected in some cases. A mother's physical incapacity could result in a child becoming a carer: being a child carer brings a burden that may be unbearable. One symphysiotomy mother relates how, four years ago, after a lifetime of looking after her, her son took his own life. Such a tragedy illustrates how the *sequelae*, as doctors term it, of one potentially crippling operation may carry through the generations.

For women who were particularly badly damaged, the operation led to a lifetime of loss. Being unable to participate fully in significant family events, such as First Communion, left its mark. Aileen McNamara explains that she was unable to attend any family occasions or functions: 'I took panic attacks … All my young years and family life were destroyed'. That loss is a continuing one for some. Bridget O'Sullivan underlines how the damage she sustained means 'not being able to do things I'd like to, like … having fun with my grandchildren … I couldn't play with my own children when they were young'.

The surgery, in some cases, gave rise to internal tensions within families, where the need for the operation was disputed. Husbands occasionally took refuge in denial, as did other family members. Siblings and others sometimes took sides. As with abuse, the topic was often taboo. One mother said her family would not understand. 'It's a big secret. I've never been able to talk about it, even to my husband, even to my son [born by symphysiotomy]'. The silence surrounding the surgery was deafening. Even sisters were not told, in some cases, nor sisters-in-law, nor brothers, nor brothers-in-law. Nor friends. Women occasionally expressed feelings of shame and guilt: 'I would be very ashamed to tell anyone that this happened to me. It has divided families … I know what happened wasn't my fault. But I felt it was me that was to blame'.

The sundering of the pelvis destroyed lives in a myriad of ways. While some succeeded in getting on with their lives, others were not so fortunate. As with physical damage, the surgery led to different degrees of emotional distress. For some women, their inability to function like other mothers during those early weeks and months after the birth damaged their sense of themselves as mothers and led to a profound and enduring loss of self esteem. Some mothers never regained their confidence and were forced to give up their previous employment. Depression was, and is, quite common. Some have been taking medication for it for 40 years. Some women were never again able to drive a car post symphysiotomy. Chronic pain also isolates, while symptoms too embarrassing to discuss compound the isolation and the loneliness that lack of mobility brings. A number of mothers have never got over the trauma of their operation: every day, they think about what was done to them in the labour ward or the operating theatre. Being subjected to surgery without consent, not knowing why a symphysiotomy was carried out instead of a Caesarean section, adds to the torment.

**Effects on children**

Finally, although infant morbidity [sickness] is not a subject that features in the medical literature on the surgery, there are children whose lives have been made more difficult by symphysiotomy. Depression, for example, is not uncommon among these children: their mothers tend to link it to their traumatic births. Several of these now adult children born by symphysiotomy have themselves undergone or will undergo surgery. Their mothers attribute their medical problems to the pelvis-cutting procedure. Bernadette O'Brien takes a similar view: '[My daughter] Alice was born brain damaged after the symphysiotomy and that was a life sentence for us both. It breaks my heart that she can't learn or work and is still attending a special school. She is 49 years old now and I am always blaming myself, thinking if I didn't have that operation she would be perfect. They could have done a section.'

# II 'A tragedy, not a melodrama': the official view

*'The real story [of symphysiotomy] is more complex - a tragedy, not a melodrama.'*

Peter Boylan and Tony Farmer.[60]

## Omerta

The practice of symphysiotomy, while reported in hospital reports, appears to have been shrouded in considerable secrecy in the clinical setting, so far as staff-patient communications were concerned. Consultant obstetricians reportedly neglected to inform mothers in advance of their surgery, while midwives often omitted to explain to their patients why they were in such pain after childbirth. Mothers were often also at a loss to know why their babies were in intensive care, and why they were denied access to them.

The Harding Clark Report paints a vivid picture of *omerta* at the Lourdes Hospital, for example. The inquiry found 'a incredibly pervasive culture of acceptance and acquiescence of consultant activity'[61]. For decades, the judge recounts, senior and junior doctors in obstetrics and anaesthesia voiced no concerns about so-called Caesarean hysterectomies, nor did senior or junior midwives or nurses. Survivors of symphysiotomy have recounted how these operations were often performed during labour under the gaze of large numbers of staff. Two generations of midwives and doctors in the Lourdes, the National Maternity and the Coombe must have stood and watched as obstetricians sundered women's symphises or split their pubic bones.

---

[60] Peter Boylan and Tony Farmer 1999 'Obstetrics and Ethics' Letter *Irish Times* 6 Oct.
[61] Maureen Harding Clark 2006 *The Lourdes Hospital Inquiry An Inquiry into peripartum hysterectomy at Our Lady of Lourdes Hospital Drogheda Report of Judge Maureen Harding Clark SC.* Stationary Office, Dublin, 155.

A few general practitioners were reported to have witnessed these operations being performed on their patients in Drogheda. None subsequently came forward to complain, it appears, possibly because of the deference induced by specialisation.

Staff who did not see these operations firsthand in these hospitals must have known about them. Labour ward midwives at the Lourdes Hospital collected copious data on births, including 'deviations', on a daily basis. These statistics must have included symphysiotomy, which was mostly performed in the labour ward. Totted up at the end of each month, these figures were prominently pinned on the notice board in the nurses' station for all to read. Like other surgical procedures, symphysiotomy must have been recorded in ward daybooks, maternity theatre registers, patients' charts, clinical reports, student notebooks and, possibly, public health nurse 'books'.[62] Every midwife and every doctor on the postnatal wards would have been aware of every patient who had had her pelvis sundered. Medical record keeping at NMH and the Coombe is unlikely to have been very different: these hospitals published copious statistics in a similar format. Staff therefore who did not witness these operations in these Dublin hospitals must have been aware of the practice of surgically dividing the pelvis.

**Regulatory failure**
Detailed data on symphysiotomy were published in these hospitals' annual or bi-annual clinical reports. Even the most extreme symphysiotomies, those done in the aftermath of Caesarean section, for example, were described and tabulated in detail in the Lourdes Hospital reports.

Regulatory authorities and medical trainers ignored this evidence of what was evidently, by the accepted standards of good practice of the time, unprecedented and bizarre surgery. These clinical reports were sent to medical authorities, such as the Institute of Obstetricians and Gynaecologists, as the Medical Missionaries of Mary underlined in 2010,[63] when they issued an apology to survivors. A glance at the

---

[62] Maureen Harding Clark 2006 op cit, 127-35.
[63] Fiona Magennis 2010 'Nuns Apology' *Drogheda Independent* 24 Feb.

Lourdes report would have revealed the practice: symphysiotomy appeared in the table of contents as late as 1984.[64] The Lourdes Hospital maternity unit, under the tutelage of Dr Michael Neary, ceased to produce clinical reports in 1984.[65] This departure from established practice went unremarked, it appears. Medical trainers, such as the Royal College of Obstetrics and Gynaecology (RCOG) and the Institute of Obstetricians and Gynaecologists, whose role was not only to represent its members and advise in matters of education and training but to promote 'excellence in the areas of patient care, [and] professional standards'[66] continued to accredit these hospitals for training in obstetrics.

**Exposé**

The latter-day practice of symphysiotomy in Ireland was first exposed by a historian in a national newspaper in 1999.[67] Dr Jacqueline Morrissey was completing a doctoral thesis at University College Dublin on the relationship between the Catholic Church and the medical profession in Ireland. Tracing the impact of this relationship on the practice of obstetrics and gynaecology,[68] she discovered the latter-day practice of symphysiotomy in Dublin. Writing in the *Irish Times*, she highlighted the dangers of the surgery, describing in detail the storm of controversy provoked by its revival at NMH, and concluded that the operation was religiously motivated. This article drew fire from a former Master of the National Maternity, Dr Peter Boylan and his brother-in-law, Holles St historian, Tony Farmar.[69] They contended that 'symphysiotomy was driven not by Catholic teaching but by the medical risks associated with repeated Cesareans' [sic], an argument previously

---

64 *Our Lady of Lourdes Hospital Drogheda International Missionary Training Centre Clinical Report* Maternity Department 1984: 32.
65 Maureen Harding Clark 2006 op cit, 274.
66 Institute of Obstetricians and Gynaecologists 2010 'Statement on symphysiotomy'. 17 Feb.
67 Jacqueline Morrisey 1999 'Midwifery of Darker Times' *Irish Times* 6 Sept.
68 Jacqueline K Morrisey 2004 *An examination of the relationship between the Catholic Church and the medical profession in Ireland in the period 1922 – 1992, with particular emphasis on the impact of this relationship in the field of reproductive medicine*. Unpublished PhD thesis University College Dublin.
69 Peter Boylan and Tony Farmer 1999 op cit.

Bodily Harm | 37

made by former NMH Masters. Repeat Caesareans, according to Boylan and Farmar, had mortal implications in a culture where large families were the norm, as doctors had a duty to respect their patients' beliefs. A 1993 text co-authored by Boylan put forward the idea that symphysiotomy had been revived at Holles St 'to offset the commitment to repeat caesarean sections in young mothers with a diagnosis of cephalopelvic disproportion'.[70] The notion of *a commitment* to repeat Caesarean section was predicated on the idea of a culture where family limitation was unknown.

---

**4. Myths and red herrings**
'Symphysiotomy was an obstetrical procedure used by clinicians during the 1940s, 1950s and 1960s....This procedure was used in an era when Caesarean sections carried a higher risk to the mother.' Dr Moffatt, Minister for State at the Department of Health, 2001. [71]

---

**IOG defence**
Following Jacqueline Morrissey's exposé of the practice, the Chief Medical Officer of the Department of Health sought a report on symphysiotomy from the Institute of Obstetricians and Gynaecologists, some of whose members or former members had carried out these operations. On 4 May 2001, the Institute responded with a one-page letter, thereafter officially referred to as a 'report' (See Appendix 1). The IOG's central point was that symphysiotomy was the norm for obstructed labour until the 1950s, when antibiotics became available and symphysiotomy was *replaced* by Caesarean section. Dr Moffatt, Minister for State at the Department of Health, had already told the Dáil one day earlier that symphysiotomy was used in an era when Caesarean sections carried a higher risk to the mother.[72] A health board 'information leaflet' later specified that this era was 'between the 1950's and the 1980's'.

---

[70] Kieran O Driscoll, Declan Meagher with Peter Boylan 1993 *Active Management of Labor The Dublin Experience* 3rd ed. Mosby, London, 65.
[71] Dr Tom Moffatt TD 2001 *Dáil Debates* Adjournment Debate Hospital Practices Vol 535 No 3 Col 987-8 3 May .
[72] Ibid

The Institute's letter has been used as the basis of all ministerial and departmental statements on symphysiotomy for the past decade.[73, 74, 75, 76, 77, 78] The IOG described the operation as 'permanently enlarging the pelvis', omitting to mention that this enlargement was achieved by severing the symphysis or cutting the pubic bone. Mistakenly, the Institute told the Department of Health that symphysiotomy was carried out *mainly* in the National Maternity and the Coombe Hospitals from 1920 to 1960. An image of maternal death was invoked, with women presenting in hospital as emergencies in obstructed labour, at risk of dying in a pre-antibiotic era from infection, should a Caesarean section be undertaken. Wrongly, the IOG contended that symphysiotomy was the norm for obstructed labour until the 1950s, when antibiotics became available and symphysiotomy was *replaced* by Caesarean section. 'Excellent results' had been 'claimed' for the procedure, the letter said, adding that, 'in properly conducted cases, complications were rare'.

While symphysiotomy has been repeatedly portrayed by the authorities in Ireland as a life-saving operation, performed solely for medical reasons, that was safe for mothers and babies, Irish obstetrics has shown itself to be divided on the issue. While the IOG has always maintained that symphysiotomy was the norm for obstructed labour, this claim has been disputed. Dr Boylan, a leading member of the Institute, has publicly stated that Caesarean section was the standard treatment for obstructed labour.[79] There is also fundamental disagreement on another critical point: the complication for which symphysiotomy was performed. In a letter defending the practice of

---

[73] Micheál Martin TD 2001 *Dáil Debates* Written Answers Maternity Services Vol 541 No 3 Col 930 4 Oct.

[74] Micheál Martin TD 2003 *Dáil Debates* Written Answers Maternity Services Vol 567 No 2 Col 542-3 21 May.

[75] Brian Lenihan TD 2002 *Dáil Debates* Hospital Practices Vol 567 No 5 Col 1008-9 27 May.

[76] Micheál Martin TD 2003 *Dáil Debates* Surgical Procedures Vol 569 No 3 Col 339-40 24 June.

[77] Micheál Martin TD 2003 *Dáil Debates* Written Answers Maternity Services Vol 569 Col 932 25 June.

[78] Darragh Scully, Private Secretary to the Minister for Health and Children 2009. Letter to the Joint Committee on Health. Oct.

[79] Peter Boylan and Tony Farmer 1999 'Obstetrics and Ethics' Letter *Irish Times* 6 Oct.

symphysiotomy in the medical press in 2010, former IOG Chairman, Dr Conor Carr, claimed that disproportion was common in Ireland,[80] while Dr Peter Boylan is on record as saying disproportion did not exist[81] and that the practice of symphysiotomy was unnecessary.

**Delayed discovery of an operation**
Many of those who had been symphysiotomised first learned of their surgery through the media. It played a critical role, not only in bringing symphysiotomy to public attention, but in bringing these operations to private notice. Many women were discharged from hospital without knowing that their pelvises had been broken. Some survivors in the East learned about their surgery three  or four decades later, after reading about symphysiotomy in an evening newspaper.[82, 83] Matilda Behan, who was featured in these articles, set up  a support group with the help of her daughter, Bernadette, and the newly formed Survivors of Symphysiotomy launched in Dublin in May 2002, under the aegis of the National Women's Council of Ireland.[84] The meeting, which was packed to capacity, was addressed by John Gormley TD and Senator Mary Henry, among others, all of whom pledged support for SoS.

Casualties of the surgery in the North-East discovered that they had been symphysiotomised when LMFM's Paul Maguire broadcast interviews in 2002 with former patients of the Lourdes who had undergone the operation. For some, the discovery, 30 or 40 years on, that they had been symphysiotomised was deeply disturbing. Where it was done under general anaesthetic, particularly, the knowledge that their bodies had been 'invaded' without their knowledge and without their consent was overwhelming. Women felt that their sense of self had been violated.

---

[80]  Conor Carr 2010 'Symphysiotomy helped women have multiple births' Letter *Irish Medical Times* 25 March.
[81]  Peter Boylan and Tony Farmer 1999 op cit.
[82]  Carl O'Brien 2001. 'Brutal operations continued until 1975' *Irish Examiner* 20 Apr.
[83]  Isabel Hurley 2002 'Women unite in pact against barbaric ops' *Evening Herald* 10 May.
[84]  Aine O'Connor 2002 'When giving birth becomes a mother's worst nightmare' *Sunday Independent* 5 May.

> **5. Myths and red herrings**
> 'Symphysiotomy is safe for the mother from a vital perspective, confers a permanent enlargement of the pelvis and facilitates vaginal delivery in future pregnancies, and is a life saving operation for the child. Severe complications are rare.' Dr Kenneth Bjorklund, 2002.[85]

## Dr Kenneth Bjorklund

SoS's campaign for an independent inquiry gave rise to a further burst of artillery from NMH. Writing once again in the *Irish Times*, Dr Boylan quoted a Swedish obstetrician[86] in support of his contention that symphysiotomy was as safe as Caesarean section.[87] This was the first assertion in the national media that symphysiotomy was safe for mothers. The former NMH Master asserted that, while the rate of long-term complications was 'the same' for both operations, the death rate for mothers was six times higher following Caesarean section. No cases of walking difficulty had been identified despite long-term follow-up of symphysiotomy cases, he said.

Dr Kenneth Bjorklund, the Swedish author quoted by Dr Boylan, had written a review of all the studies published on symphysiotomy in the 20th century, with a view to compiling statistics to demonstrate the value of the surgery in developing countries. Bjorklund's work, which is written from a pro-symphysiotomy perspective, has been widely used to support the view that symphysiotomy is safe for mothers by those who seek to defend its latter day practice in Ireland. However, while his article is of historical interest, his statistics are both invalid and unreliable.

An examination of Bjorklund's review reveals that its evidential value was extremely limited and that very little was known, scientifically,

---

[85] Kenneth Bjorklund 2002 'Minimally invasive surgery for obstructed labour: a review of symphysiotomy during the twentieth century (including 5000 cases)'. *British Journal of Obstetrics and Gynaecology* 109 (3): 236-48.

[86] Ibid.

[87] Peter Boylan 2003 'Symphysiotomy and Caesarean section' Letter *Irish Times* 17 June.

about the surgery. Dr Jacqueline Morrissey has drawn attention to such aspects as the dubious value of reports compiled in the early part of the twentieth century whose methodological defects were glaring.[88] Like was not being compared with like in the compilation of Bjorklund's statistics: problems of definition were ignored. One medical author counted 'walking difficulties' on the seventh day following surgery, for example, while another enumerated them after four weeks and what constituted walking difficulties, in any event, was not defined. Also, surgery became safer as the century progressed: there was little or no comparison between the safety of the 'classic' Caesarean section in 1910 and that of the 'lower segment' Caesarean 50 years later. All formed the basis of Bjorklund's statistics, however. There were also problems of professional, cultural and gender bias (see Appendix II). Seen from outside obstetrics, the specialty's view of what ought to be viewed as injurious appeared to be very narrow. Obstetricians tended to understate the side effects of the surgery, focusing on fetal deaths, for example, and ignoring fetal injuries.

Moreover, what doctors knew about symphysiotomy was largely based on small to minuscule numbers that would not be acceptable according to generally held statistical standards. Bjorklund's 2002 statistics were compiled using 'studies' that consisted of as few as four cases, although just over 1 000 are required for research to be considered statistically significant. Adding the results of these small to minuscule studies together to generate new statistics gave rise to further problems, with the lack of comparability between disparate bits and pieces of research adding to the general invalidity and unreliability of Bjorklund's results. The problem of low numbers was even more marked in research relating to the surgery's side effects. With obstetricians studying the long-term effects of their handiwork in just 129 women over a period of 100 years,[89] the surgery's consequences were virtually unknown. Bjorklund cited just three long-term follow up studies, all of them statistically defective, before concluding erroneously that symphysiotomy was safe for mothers. 'There is considerable evidence

---

[88] Jacqueline K Morrisey 2004 op cit, 180.
[89] Kenneth Bjorklund 2002 op cit.

to support a reinstatement of symphysiotomy in the obstetric arsenal, for the benefit of women in obstructed labour and their offspring' he asserted, an argument that is clearly unsustainable on the basis of his own description of the utterly inadequate statistics used in compiling this 'evidence'.

On 1 October 2003, the then Minister for Health, Micheál Martin, promised an external 'review' of the surgery.[90] Having first looked to the Institute of Obstetricians for 'guidance', the Department of Health requested Dr Bjorklund to review the latterday practice of symphysiotomy in Ireland. SoS objected to his nomination upon learning of his partiality for the operation, and he subsequently withdrew from the process, citing 'pressure of work.'[91] Martin's successor, Mary Harney, used Bjorklund's withdrawal to terminate the proposed review, citing 'difficulties in sourcing a reviewer'. Since then, the authorities have maintained that only those who have published on symphysiotomy in the medical press could be deemed suitable to review the practice in Ireland. However, almost all the articles published on the surgery in the literature are authored by tropical doctors generally intent on presenting the results of their own symphysiotomies in a favourable light. In January 2006, Ms Harney extended a surprise personal invitation to the then Chairperson of SoS to a meeting attended by herself and three senior functionaries. The official view, namely, that an external review would be of 'no benefit', was, according to Department of Health minutes of the meeting, allegedly 'agreed.'[92]

## The Lourdes Inquiry

The Lourdes Hospital first came to public notice when a national newpaper revealed that a number of Caesarean hysterectomies judged to be unnecessary had been carried out at its maternity unit. Several doctors at the hospital had a tendency to remove women's wombs following Caesarean section. Also, women occasionally woke up from

---

[90] http://www.rte.ie/news/2003/1001/symphyisotomy.html
[91] Carl O'Brien 2004 'Expert to review 'barbaric' surgery backed procedure' *Irish Times* 19 July
[92] Department of Health and Children 2006 Minutes of SoS meeting with Minister for Health, among others. 17 Jan.

a general anaesthetic to find that their uterus had been removed during treatment for a miscarriage, for example, or a delayed placenta. Women's ovaries, singly and in pairs, were also removed. Nearly all of these operations — which rendered women infertile — were unnecessary, it transpired. From 1974-1998, of the women who underwent a Caesarean section there, 188 had their wombs removed immediately afterwards, or shortly thereafter. While the rate of Caesarean hysterectomy at the hospital was 20 times higher than in other hospitals, nothing was done for a quarter of a century to protect women against involuntary sterilisation.

In September 2003, a group representing the casualties, Patient Focus, asked the government to set up a statutory public inquiry into the functioning of the Lourdes maternity unit[93] from 1974 onwards. This proposal effectively precluded any investigation of the many symphysiotomies carried out in Drogheda in earlier decades. Yet the Lourdes  had already been exposed as an epicentre, not only of Caesarean hysterectomy, but also of symphysiotomy.[94] Referring to the practice of breaking the pelvis in childbirth, Sinn Fein TD Arthur Morgan told the Dáil in June 2003 that 'what these women suffered [at the Lourdes] is on a par with institutional abuse.'[95]

In the event, the government refused to hold a statutory public inquiry of any kind into the hospital, opting instead for a narrow private inquiry into the practice of what it termed 'peripartum hysterectomy'. The inquiry's terms of reference excluded ovariotomies, symphysiotomies and even some hysterectomies. Thereafter, the focus of the inquiry narrowed even further, highlighting the role of Dr Michael Neary, who had already been struck off by the Medical Council for malpractice, for example, and leaving colleagues at the maternity unit who had engaged in similar practices largely uninvestigated.

---

93  Sheila O'Connor 2010 *Without Consent The Dr Michael Neary Nightmare The story of almost 200 women damaged by one doctor.* Poolbeg, Dublin, 290.
94  Fintan O'Toole 2003 'Michael Neary and butchering women'. *Irish Times* 8 May.
95  Arthur Morgan TD 2003 *Dáil Debates* Other Questions Surgical Procedures Vol 569 Col 343 24 June.

## Human Rights Commission

Hopes that the Irish Human Rights Commission might carry out its own review into symphysiotomy were subsequently dashed. Patient Focus, which by then had become a patient advocacy service, asked the Commission to investigate the issue under Section 9 (1) (b) of the Human Rights Commission Act 2000, but it declined to do so, partly on the basis of the 'very useful' information supplied to it in October 2007 by the Department of Health, which was probably based on the IOG's 2001 letter. In October 2008, however, for reasons that are not known, the Commission changed its view and formally advised the Government, this time under Section 8 (d) of the Act, to reconsider its decision not to review symphysiotomy. The Minister for Health declined to accept the Commission's advice. Survivors of symphysiotomy, together with SoS's legal advisor, Colm MacGeehin, met members of the Joint Oireachtas Committee on Health and Children in June 2009. Following the *in camera* meeting, the Joint Committee unanimously recommended an independent inquiry into the surgery. In response, Minister for Health Mary Harney declined to set up even a review.

### *Prime Time*

A *Prime Time Special* on the issue on 18 February 2010 and watched by over 400,000 viewers, scandalised the nation, with harrowing testimony from survivors interwoven with expert comment. Journalist Paul Maguire revealed that 1500 of these operations had been performed, far in excess of the 600 that had hitherto been uncovered. Viewers were left in no doubt that the surgery had been impelled by religious motives, training needs and medical experimentation. The IOG issued a lengthy statement[96] (see Appendix 3) the day before the broadcast that, once again, was non-specific as to when and where symphysiotomy had been performed, effectively veiling time periods and geographic locations. Suggesting that symphysiotomy was done for medical reasons, the Institute claimed that 'the procedure also offered the prospect of safer vaginal delivery in future pregnancies at a time when large family size

---

[96]   Institute of Obstetricians and Gynaecologists 2010 Statement on Symphysiotomy 17 Feb.

was usual'. Reiterating its 2001 position, the IOG claimed that symphysiotomy was 'simpler and safer' than Caesarean section, an operation that 'gradually replaced' it during the 20th century. (The idea that symphysiotomy was replaced by Caesarean section in Ireland in the 1950s can also be found on the web site of Patient Focus, where this myth is presented as though it were a fact.[97]) Citing the Bjorklund article, the IOG statement suggested that problems, such as walking difficulties, pelvic pain and urinary incontinence, might be expected to resolve within six months maximum.

### Carte blanche

The day after the *Prime Time* programme aired, the Minister for Health and Children ruled out any investigation of symphysiotomy, saying that, 'as symphysiotomy was superseded by Caesarean section in the *1980s* [my italics], any review would not now be productive'.[98] Four days later, the junior minister at her Department, John Moloney TD, announced that Minister Harney had asked the Institute of Obstetricians and Gynaecologists to prepare its own report on the practice.[99] The IOG was given *carte blanche* to draw up its own terms of reference, as none were suggested to guide its report. Indeed, the Minister's letter was notable for its lack of specificity as to the period of time and geographic location(s) to be covered by the report. In her letter, she requested 'that the report would provide the Institute's assessment of the circumstances in which symphysiotomy was carried out in Irish obstetric units; indicate what protocols or guidance existed over the years to guide professional practice; specify when the practice changed and why it changed at that time in Ireland'. Patient Focus welcomed the review.

These formulations clearly loaded the dice in respect of the report sought, however. For the Minister to ask for an assessment of the circumstances under which symphysiotomy was carried out might evoke a defence of the surgery, grounded in such ideas as the Catholic view of birth control, and

---

[97] http://patientfocus.ie/site/index.php/patientfocus/cases/symphysiotomy/
[98] http://www.rte.ie/news/2010/0219/symphysiotomy.html.
[99] John Moloney TD 2010 *Dáil Debates* Adjournment Debate Hospital Procedures Vol 703 No 1 Col 85-6 23 Feb.

buttressed by such notions as the over-whelming trend towards large families, the widespread prevalence of malnutrition, the common occurrence of rickets, the large numbers of contracted pelvises, and so forth. The request to specify the protocols guiding symphysiotomy might also result in some justification for the surgery on the basis that no protocols were available during those decades to inform medical practice. Finally, asking the IOG to specify when and why the practice of symphysiotomy 'changed' implied that, as per the Institute's own fanciful theory, symphysiotomy was the norm in Ireland for difficult births until it was overtaken by Caesarean section. This is a claim that is without the slightest foundation, as is shown in Chapter IV.

The day after John Moloney's announcement of an internal inquiry by the IOG, Fianna Fáil's Geraldine Feeney, who had sat for three years on the fitness to practice inquiry into Michael Neary's practice of involuntary sterilisation at the Lourdes, told the Senate: 'this matter [symphysiotomy] cannot be left to the small cosy cartel that is the Institute of Obstetricians and Gynaecologists'.[100] However, the Minister for Health — and presumably, her Department — disagreed: in her opinion, the rightness or wrongness of the latter day practice of symphysiotomy was a question for the Institute. 'As an obstetric procedure, it [symphysiotomy] is, and has been, a matter primarily for the Institute of Obstetricians and Gynaecologists to advise and lead upon'.[101] The government's view was repeated on 20 April.[102]

SoS reiterated its demand for an independent inquiry, on the basis that commissioning the Institute to undertake a report on symphysiotomy amounted to a self-review. These operations, SoS argued, were carried out by IOG members or former members, took place in hospitals where IOG members work or worked, and were likely approved for training purposes by the IOG (and its predecessor, the RCOG). Labour Party TD Jan O Sullivan (now Minister of State for Trade) challenged

---

[100] Geraldine Feeney 2010 *Seanad Debates* Order of Business Col 201 No 2 Col 68-9 24 Feb.

[101] Mary Harney TD 2010 *Dáil Debates* Written answers 'Medical Inquiries' Vol 703 No 3 Col 622-3 25 Feb.

[102] Mary Harney TD 2010 *Dáil Debates* Written answers Medical Procedures Vol 706 No 3 Col 598 20 Apr.

the Minister's view that the IOG was an appropriate body to review the surgery: 'my questions relate to the fact that a body which is directly implicated, namely, the Institute of Obstetricians and Gynaecologists, has been appointed to examine this matter.'[103]

**Sallies and defences**
The *Prime Time* programme led to other sallies in defence of the operation, centering on the absurd proposition that doctors were saving women from the theoretical risk of dying from repeat Caesarean sections by physically sundering their pelvises. Writing in the *Irish Times*, Dr John McCarthy, a retired anaesthetist, highlighted the aetiology of the contracted pelvis, the absence of sterilisation and contraception, the mortal dangers of repeat Caesarean section and the infrequency of gait problems following symphysiotomy.[104] A former Chairman of the IOG, Dr Conor Carr, made similar points in the medical press, again predicated on the idea that (during four decades of symphysiotomy practice) family planning was not a option,[105] another baseless contention, as demonstrated in Chapter IV.

The IOG had been asked by the Minister to complete its report by the end of April 2010: no report issued, however. Two months after the deadline had expired, the Minister told the Dáil the Institute was 'finalising' a team to write its report. Some details of the team, revealed to the Joint Health Committee four days later, afterwards appeared in the medical press.[106]

Subsequent engagement with the IOG revealed draft terms of reference (see Appendix 4) that, like the Minister's letter, lacked specificity as to period and place and could be seen to hark back to the Institute's 2010 statement and its 2001 letter. Unlike those drawn up by the Harding

---

[103] Jan O'Sullivan TD 2010 *Dáil Debates* Order of Business Vol 705 No 3 Col 522 25 March.
[104] John R McCarthy 2010 'Controversy over childbirth operation' Letter *Irish Times* 1 March.
[105] Conor Carr 2010 'Symphysiotomy helped women have multiple births' Letter *Irish Medical Times* 25 March.
[106] Gary Culliton 2010 'Symphysiotomy report is due within months.' *Irish Medical News* 20 Aug.

Clark Inquiry, the Institute's terms specified no time frame, suggesting that the revival of symphysiotomy in Ireland in 1944 might be left unexamined. Neither did they refer to Caesarean section, so whether or not this operation enjoyed medical approval during those decades, and, if so, whether or not doctors opted to carry out a symphysiotomy instead, might, on the face of it, be left unexamined. One term of reference, which asked 'when the practice changed and why', seemed to suggest that symphysiotomy, during a relevant period, was the treatment of choice for difficult births, again an unsustainable proposition. Finally, the IOG's terms made no mention of survivors' injuries, implying that the operation's long-term consequences might not be assessed.

## Potential conflicts of interest

Further potential conflict of interest issues arose. The IOG's report writing team was to be chaired by Dr James Dornan,[107] an eminent professor at Queen's University and a former International Vice-Chair of the RCOG, the representative body for the specialty in Ireland in the 1940s, 50s and 60s, to which those responsible for these operations belonged. (Since the 1970s, Irish obstetricians, North and South, have held dual membership of both the RCOG and the IOG.) The RCOG had, and has, business interests in symphysiotomy: it publishes and sells training manuals that include instructions on how to perform it.[108] Symphysiotomy is taught as part of an RCOG course in emergency obstetrics in London[109] and these courses are taught across Britain[110] by instructors who presumably include RCOG members.

The IOG planned to commission a literature review of symphysiotomy from the Liverpool School of Tropical Medicine. This review, to be paid for with public monies, was to form the centrepiece of the Institute's report for the Minister. Dr Nynke van den Broek, a leading proponent of symphysiotomy, who advocates that it be taught as a core skill to

---

[107] Ibid.
[108] Charlotte Howell, Kate Grady and Charles Cox 2007 *Managing Obstetric Emergencies and Trauma – the MOET Course Manual*. 2nd ed. RCOG, London.
[109] Institute of Obstetricians and Gynaecologists 2010 op cit.
[110] http://www.alsg.org.

'skilled birth attendants' in developing countries,[111] was selected by the IOG to take charge of this literature review. It subsequently emerged that van den Broek and Dornan had led the setting up of a consortium on behalf of their respective institutions to teach skilled birth attendance in developing countries. Since 2006, that partnership has brought business opportunities from all over the world for both the Royal College and the Liverpool School.[112]

**Tropical literature**
The value of the IOG's proposed literature review to Irish survivors was unclear. Moreover, symphysiotomy had been reported almost exclusively in Africa in the second half of the last century: the review would inevitably examine the practice of symphysiotomy in Ireland through the lens of medicine as practiced in Africa. This was not an appropriate context in which to frame an examination of the surgery in Ireland. There were also legitimate concerns in relation to inherent bias, as any study of the literature on symphysiotomy was bound to conclude in its favour. Those tropical doctors writing about symphysiotomy tend to favour the practice, as they are invariably presenting the results of their own handiwork. Also, these studies did not generally reveal the long-term consequences of the surgery, partly because their authors were persuaded that symphysiotomy was safe for mothers, and partly because not enough patients had ever been followed up for long enough.

The IOG refused to amend its draft terms of reference or to abandon its plans to commission a literature review from the Liverpool School of Tropical Medicine. SoS's proposal that survivors' injuries should be quantified, medically, and that the wider fall-out from the surgery should be studied, systematically, was rejected: the IOG's plans to 'meet

---

[111] AA Adegoke and N Van Den Broek 2009 'Skilled birth attendance-lessons learnt'. *British Journal of Obstetrics and Gynaecology* Special Issue: International Reviews Oct 116: 33-40.
[112] Royal College of Obstreticians and Gynaecologists 2006. Setting standards to improve womens health Annual Report and Financial Statements. RCOG, London, 29

and greet' survivors in batches and invite them to tell their 'stories' in group settings remained unaltered.

These concerns were conveyed to the Department of Health. SoS proposals for a Bristol-style inquiry,[113] including draft terms of reference (see Appendix 5), and suggested experts in law, sociology and history yielded only a brief, non-committal response from a deputy chief medical officer. The IOG was seeking £30,000 from the Department to carry out its tropical literature review. SoS queried the use of public monies to hire the Liverpool School and suggested that public funds would be better spent on a study of the surgery's long-term side effects. No interest was shown in this proposal or in the idea that there might be potential conflicts of interest or inherent bias in *any* review of the tropical literature. It seemed clear that whatever the Institute was planning had the support of the Department of Health.

**A change of plan**
At a general meeting in December 2010, SoS took a decision not to co-operate with the Institute's plans, on the basis they were unlikely to uncover the truth about these operations. Three committee members disagreed with the otherwise unanimous decision of the members, however. A prominent article in a national newspaper exposing some of the conflicts of interest[114] subsequently led to an unspecified change of plan on the part of the Institute. This was announced to the media by Patient Focus, who expressed disappointment that the IOG review was not now going ahead as planned. A company calling itself Survivors of Symphysiotomy Ltd was subsequently registered in March 2011: the memorandum was signed by three former SoS committee members and by three staff members of Patient Focus. The business address of the HSE-funded patient service Provider was given as the administrative address of Survivors of Symphysiotomy Ltd. IOG subsequently informed the Department of Health that communications were to go to a representative of Survivors of Symphysiotomy Ltd.[115]

---

[113] http://www.bristol-inquiry.org.uk.
[114] Carl O'Brien 2010 'Report on "brutal"childbirth surgery will be flawed, claims survivors' group' *Irish Times* 21 Oct.
[115] Mark Costigan 2011. Email to Olivia Kearney 16 May.

Little information has been released on what the Institute is now planning. Over a year after the deadline for the IOG's original report, it is not known whether the IOG's initial report writing team is still in place, or whether the tropical literature review is going ahead. Three Dáil questions have failed to clarify these issues. The first[116] elucidated the information that 'alternative arrangements' involving 'a university school of public health' were being made. Despite being asked to do so, the Minister gave no information on the overall IOG report or its contents, the composition of the team, or the new deadline, if any. Ms Harney's successors answered in similarly vague terms. [117a, 117b]

It later transpired that a historian from University College Cork had been commissioned by the Chief Medical Officer, on foot of a request by the Minister for Health, James Reilly, and following 'discussions' with the Institute and 'patient groups' to draw up a report on symphysiotomy[118]. The same defective terms of reference as those given by Mary Harney to the IOG, will govern this review, namely, to assess the circumstances in which symphysiotomy was carried out; indicate what protocols existed at the time; and specify when the practice changed and why.[119] The latter term, particularly, dovetails with the idea that symphysiotomy was 'gradually replaced by Caesarean section [in Ireland] as the preferred method of delivery', as Kathleen Lynch TD, Minister of State at the Department of Health, told the Dáil.[120] The briefing note provided to the new Minister by the Department of Health states that 'little if any new learning would be gained from a full-scale inquiry'.[121]

---

[116] Mary Harney TD 2011 *Dáil Debates* Department of Health and Children Medical Reports Written answers Vol 726 No 2 Col 635 13 Jan.

[117a] Mary Coughlan TD 2011 *Dáil Debates* Department of Health and Children Medical Reviews Written answers Vol 727 No 5 Col 881 27 Jan.

[117b] Dr James Reilly TD 2011 *Dáil Debates* Written Answers Hospital Procedures Vol 728 No 5 24 March.

[118] Jennifer Martin 2011 Email to Tom Moran 12 May

[119] Danielle Barron 2011 'Symphysiotomy report to be carried out'. *Irish Medical News* 23 May.

[120] Kathleen Lynch TD 2011 *Dáil Debates* Hospital Procedures Vol 730 No 4 Col 721-2 20 Apr.

[121] Danielle Barron 2011 op cit.

# III 'If we were a load of men': health and disability issues

*If we were a load of men, we'd have got on a lot better!*
Vera Kennedy, a survivor of symphysiotomy.

Symphysiotomy survivors face a very wide range of health problems today as a result of their surgery. Despite a general worsening with age of their condition, women's access to appropriate and comprehensive health care, free of charge, is being increasingly restricted. Essential medical needs, ranging, potentially, from pelvic surgery to pain relief, are not being met in some cases. Many women have to pay for medical or other treatments and/or supplies that are supposed to be provided free of charge by the state to casualties of the surgery. Contrary to official claims, no comprehensive package is in place today to meet their health care needs. Preliminary results of an SoS survey show that many of the benefits and entitlements promised by the former Government in 2003 have been reduced or, in some cases, withdrawn. Access to services is, and has been, a postcode lottery. Many survivors reside in the North-East, while others are clustered in Dublin, the South and South-East. The North-East seems to have been been somewhat better served than other regions, reflecting, perhaps, the younger age profile of survivors and their greater energy. In other parts of the country, where women tend to be older, their relative inability to pursue a recalcitrant bureaucracy has led to a double, or even treble, discrimination, with age combining with disability and geography to ensure that rhose most in need are often least looked after.

General practitioners have a critical role to play in ensuring women's access to appropriate health care free of charge. However the refusal of some health professionals to accept that the health problems  women present with today may be related to the surgery is a potent barrier to diagnosis and treatment. Veronica Garland explained why she had to pay for a bone scan herself: 'my doctor would not send me about my back pain, and shoulders and feet and hands. He kept saying it was wear and tear'. While survivors who complain of chronic pain are no longer dismissed out of hand, there is no doubting the widespread lack of understanding, or resistance, to the idea of the surgery's possible side effects. Witness the survivor in the West who visited her general practitioner in spring 2010 with a view to arranging a pelvic x-ray: her doctor contacted a number of private and public health care facilities, only to be told, wrongly, that symphysiotomy would certainly not be visible on x-ray. An information leaflet from an unidentified health board to general practitioners and pharmacists reportedly failed to issue.

---

**6. Myths and red herrings**
'The women concerned continue to receive attention and care through a number of services which have been put in place including: the provision of medical cards to all Survivors of Symphysiotomy (SOS) patients who requested them, the nomination, since 2003, of a Liaison Officer for a patients' group comprised of women who underwent a symphysiotomy procedure, the availability of independent clinical advice for former patients by Liaison Officers who assist in co-ordinating the provision of services to those patients, the organisation of individual pathways of care and the arrangement of appropriate follow-up, including Medical Assessment, Gynaecology Assessment, Orthopaedic Assessment, Counselling, Physiotherapy, Reflexology, Home Help, Acupuncture, Osteopathy and fast tracked hospital appointments, the refund of medical expenses related to symphysiotomy in respect of medication/private treatments, the establishment of a triple assessment service for patients at Cappagh Hospital, Dublin in January 2005, and a Support Group facilitated by a counsellor which was set up in 2004 in Dundalk and Drogheda for women living in North East region'. Mary Harney TD and Minister for Health, 2010. [122]

---

[122] Mary Harney TD 2010 *Dáil Debates* Written answers 'Medical Inquiries' Vol 715 No 2 Col 598 8 July.

The lived experience of survivors is at odds with this totalising statement, which has been repeated at intervals in the Dáil since May 2005.[123, 124,125,126,127,128,129,130,131,132,133,] most recently on 20 April 2011.[134]

Many mothers remain without access to the medical assistance and supplies that they require free of charge. Issues with medical cards have increased in the last couple of years. While all symphysiotomy casualties are entitled to a medical card, some are without one, while others live in fear of losing theirs. SoS medical cards were issued from 2003. While the exact entitlements behind these cards were never fully specified to survivors, they carried a special patient identifier to enable 'the fast-tracking of patients requiring hospital appointments and treatments' and 'the provision of certain non-GMS items'.[135] Crucially, the cards were 'for life': [136] they were also believed to offer choice of

[123] Micheál Martin TD 2004a *Dáil Debates* Written Answers Survivors of Symphysiotomy Vol 581 No 3 Col 756 3 March.

[124] Mary Harney TD 2010 *Dáil Debates* Written answers 'Hospital Services' Vol 712 No 3 Col 593-4 16 June .

[125] Mary Harney TD 2010 *Dáil Debates* Written answers 'Medical Procedures' Vol 706 No 3 Col 598 20 Apr.

[126] Mary Harney TD 2010 *Dáil Debates* Written answers 'Medical Inquiries' Vol 703 No 3 Col 622-3 25 Feb.

[127] John Moloney TD 2010 *Dáil Debates* Adjournment Debate 'Hospital Procedures' 23 Feb.

[128] Mary Harney TD 2006 *Dáil Debates* Written answers Vol 622 No 78 Col 1426-7 28 June.

[129] Mary Harney TD 2005a *Dáil Debates* Written answers 'Health Services' Vol 607 Col 1637-8 18 Oct.

[130] Mary Harney TD 2005b *Dáil Debates* Written answers 'Survivors of Symphysiotomy' Vol 602 No 5 Col 1437-8 18 May.

[131] Mary Harney TD 2005c *Dáil Debates* Written answers 'Survivors of Symphysiotomy' Vol 601 No 6 Col 1729-20 5 May.

[132] Micheál Martin TD 2004b *Dáil Debates* Written Answers 'Health Support Services' Vol 589 No 1 Col 438-9 29 Sept .

[133] Micheal Martin TD 2004a op cit.

[134] Kathleen Lynch TD 2011 *Dáil Debates* Adjournment Debate 20 'Symphysiotomy Procedures' 20 Apr. Vol 730 No 4.

[135] Mary Harney TD 2005 op cit, 2005b

[136] Angela Fitzgerald 2007 Letter to SoS members 20 Aug.

doctor. However, it is unclear whether or not the new SoS cards promised by the HSE in 2007 ever issued. Several women who were promised the old card never got it. Tellingly, all official references to special SoS medical cards have been dropped in recent years.

While expenditure on medication and private treatment relating to symphysiotomy may be refunded in theory, difficulties in obtaining reimbursement have been widely reported. One woman was forced to pay for back surgery that she could ill afford to treat the debilitating effects of symphysiotomy. Deirdre Delaney has paid for surgery to repair a prolapsed bladder. 'I could not get the treatment on the medical card'. Less well off women are now having to pay for items that were available to them free of charge two years ago. One mother has to pay for linseed oil for a bowel disorder and biofreeze for hip pain, items until recently available to her on a hardship basis. She appealed HSE's refusal of these items and six months later, was still without a reply. Many women find complementary health treatments helpful for pain control. These range from oriental therapies, such as spinal and cranial balancing, to acupuncture, osteopathy and reflexology, to name but a few. Although a number of women have had these treatments reimbursed in the past, they are being reimbursed less and less in recent years. Nuala Moriarty cannot tolerate medication very well: her family doctor recommended hydrotherapy for her back problems, but HSE said it was 'too expensive'. In another case, HSE refused to pay for acupuncture and physiotherapy. In yet another case, HSE refused to cover the cost of osteopathy for a woman who cannot now afford it, because she was widowed recently. Reimbursement for massage has also been refused. Survivors of symphysiotomy are even having to pay for services, such as chiropody and physiotherapy, that they cannot afford on their old age pensions.

Some complain of the excessive bureaucracy that refunding entails, preferring to defray the costs of medical supplies themselves. Another mother explains why, despite having a medical card, she pays for incontinence supplies herself. 'They said send in all your bills, but they make it so hard, there's always some excuse [not to pay]. It's not worth my while to claim and, to be honest, it's too embarrasssing'. Constantly changing personnel is another obstacle to reimbursement: some women have stopped applying because of this. And the requirement to keep receipts can be onerous at an age where memory may be failing. Susan O'Connell said a change of GP meant she had to pay both her doctor and her pharmacist pending the issue of her medical card: 'HSE does not seem to be aware of system for SoS...No computerised synchronisation of our hospital clinics, drugs repayments ... [There is] total confusion.'

A once off grant of €5,000 reportedly paid by Patient Focus to cover the cost of incontinence supplies remains a source of mystification, if not dissatisfaction. While a handful of survivors in the Eastern region report getting this grant, most did not, and the Dublin region was the only one in which it was disbursed. The reasons for these disparities remain unclear. Direct provision of incontinence supplies has also proved problematic, with supplies reportedly reduced in the Dublin region by 50 per cent in 2010. Although reports indicated that the HSE-supplied products were of such poor quality that they were giving rise to dermatological problems, choice of product is not generally an option.

Hardly any arrangements are in place to facilitate, co-ordinate and oversee the provision of support services to survivors. The liaison officers announced in 2003, whose job it was, among others, to organise independent clinical advice for survivors, have long vanished and some, it seems, were rarely, if ever, sighted, except in the North-East. One such officer was re-appointed by the HSE in 2010 in the North-East after a gap of several years, but no known deployment of liaison officers has occurred in other regions. These officers play a key role in ensuring access to services. Without them, women may not be aware of their entitlements, or find it difficult to negotiate the complexities of the system: they may be unable to identify relevant medical and other specialists or to secure reimbursement of medical and other fees. There are no reports of 'individual 'pathways of care' or 'fast-tracked hospital appointments', and survivor accounts suggest that they may never have existed. While a 'triple assessment' service was initiated at Cappagh Hospital, Dublin, in 2007, these gynaecological, orthopaedic and urological assessments have long since dwindled. Triple assessment required survivors to undergo a barrage of tests that included internal examinations and some older women reportedly found the concentration of these multiple assessments in a single session onerous. A similar facility for the South was mooted[137] but never materialised.

The promised telephone helpline was never implemented: the Minister for Health told the Dail it was 'agreed' to defer it.[138] The victims became the counsellors: casualties of the surgery manned a helpline themselves in 2003 following the exposure of the practice at the Lourdes Hospital on local radio, but this arrangement became unsustainable. However, that helpline was reinstated following RTE's *Prime Time* programme on symphysiotomy in February 2010. Although the surgery led to depression in some cases, no basis has been found to support the suggestion that such counselling is widely available. A small number of survivors attend monthly meetings in Drogheda run by a HSE-retained counselor. These meetings, while of benefit to participants, also enable the authorities to claim that 'counselling' is being provided, although such services are generally understood to be one-to-one.

Survivors' access to services, such as physiotherapy, reflexology, acupuncture and osteopathy, free of charge, appears to be increasingly limited. While some survivors in the North East have been able to avail of such services, they have not been reported elsewhere, even in areas with high concentrations of survivors, such as the Dublin and Cork regions.

Symphysiotomy casualties tend to suffer from mobility difficulties as well as advancing age, making housework difficult, if not impossible. Home help is perceived by them as an essential service, but contrary to official suggestions, no adequate home help service is, or has been, in place. Even in cases of marked disability, HSE assistance with housework is, and has been,[139] restricted to one or two hours per week.

---

137  Micheál Martin TD 2004 op cit, 2004b.
138  Mary Harney TD 2005 op cit, 2005c.
139  Department of Health 2006 Minutes of SoS meeting with Minister for Health, among others. 17 Jan.

In Dublin in 2010, one 84-year-old mother was offered two hours' home help per week at an out of pocket cost of €12 per hour. The service seems to be marked more by restrictions than anything else. Margaret Murray explains that her home help is 'only allowed to do light housework'. 'It's the heavy tasks, like washing windows or hanging out clothes, that I would need help with. Also, my current home help is not allowed to clean the bathroom.'

Finally, house renovations or modifications are a significant issue for women who have been particularly disabled by symphysiotomy. However, few home adaptations, if any, are being made by local authorities at the present time and awareness of the special needs and entitlements of symphysiotomy survivors appears to be low. SoS survey results to date indicate that only one respondent has succeeded in getting a bathroom grant. Eileen McArdle  was twice refused a grant by her local county council to convert her garage into a downstairs bedroom. Sarah Long says 'the house is too cold, even with insulation, which means the chronic pain becomes worse, which leads to immobility'. House improvements sought range from minor, such as the installation of stair and other rails to guard against falls, to major: renovations to enable survivors who are badly disabled to live entirely on the ground floor. Others who find the staircase difficult to negotiate simply require the installation of a stair lift.  Or bathroom facilities, such as lavatories, may need to be installed upstairs or downstairs, depending on individual wishes. One mother expressed a wish for an accessible bath 'as bending causes severe difficulty'. Many seek a walk in shower, preferably with a seat. Mary Maguire was approved such an amenity two years ago by HSE: 'I am being considered [for it] by the Borough Council...Shower approved by occupational therapist. When I enquire, I am met with great difficulty and excuses, such as cutbacks … I was promised fast tracking by the HSE but I'm still waiting'. Some survivors have reportedly been informed that disability aids, such as stair lifts and walk-in showers, are now available only to the terminally ill. Even after spinal surgery, women have reported being unable to access such essentials as grab rails and shower seats. Mary Hennessy was obliged to pay for her walk-in shower herself. Dolores Dooley also paid for a bathroom to be installed upstairs: 'I thought it hopeless to look for a grant', she says.

She would like a light, collapsible wheelchair. 'We never seem to be lucky enough to get a wheelchair in a shop. One's own would be great.'

# IV History of 'a minimally invasive surgical procedure'

*Symphysiotomy is a minimally invasive surgical procedure.*
Dr Kenneth Bjorklund, 2002.[140]

Symphysiotomy was first performed on a living woman in Paris in 1777 by a French man-midwife, Jean-René Sigault. Having failed to get a condemned criminal upon whom to experiment,[141] Sigault eventually found a woman of very small stature whom rickets had left with a contracted or deformed pelvis and who had already lost four children in childbirth. The infant survived the operation, but the mother was reportedly left with a chronic limp and a fistula, a permanent opening between the birth canal and the bladder.

---

**7. Myths and red herrings**
'The procedure [symphysiotomy] was introduced in the 18th century for selected cases of obstructed labour and proved effective in allowing vaginal births while reducing maternal and infant death and morbidity rates that related to prolonged labour. Institute of Obstetricians and Gynaecologists, 2010.[142]

---

[140] Kenneth Bjorklund 2002 Minimally invasive surgery for obstructed labour: a review of symphysiotomy during the twentieth century (including 5 000 cases). *British Journal of Obstetrics and Gynaecology* 109 (3): 236-48).

[141] F Feliciter 1895 'The History of Symphysiotomy'. *British Medical Journal* 14 Dec 1895: 1518a.

[142] Institute of Obstetricians and Gynaecologists of the Royal College of Physicians of Ireland 2010 'Statement on Symphysiotomy' 17 Feb.

Symphysiotomy was an extreme measure, performed sporadically from the late 18th century onwards at a time in when Caesarean section was viewed as unacceptably dangerous. But if Caesarean section was perceived to be high risk, symphysiotomy was very widely regarded as even more hazardous. Babies frequently died from the surgery. Mothers also died from the genital wounds inflicted upon them, while many of those who survived the surgery sustained serious and permanent side effects, among them walking difficulties and incontinence.

## A 'barbarously destructive' procedure

Published in the medical literature of the time, symphysiotomy's dismal results led to its early demise. Doctors in France bitterly disputed the merits and demerits of both Caesarean and symphysiotomy, but by the end of the 1700s, Caesarean section had won the day.[143] There was general agreement among doctors in France that, of the two procedures, Caesarean section was the safer, and the French Society of Medicine decided unanimously that doctors had a duty to carry out Caesareans. Even Sigault, before his death, repudiated the operation that had made him famous.[144]

The pelvis cutting procedure also failed to achieve respectability in these islands. So dangerous was symphysiotomy in the eyes of the medical profession that doctors refused to perform it. Dublin surgeon William Dease attacked it in 1783,[145] describing it as 'barbarously destructive', 'generally fatal to the mother and seldom successful as to saving the child'. He agreed with William Hunter's opinion that embryotomy, an operation of last resort that involved the destruction of the fetus, was preferable to symphysiotomy in cases of gross disproportion.[146] Twenty years later, Alexander Hamilton of Edinburgh

---

[143] M Baudelocque 1801 *Two Memoirs on the Caesarean operation*. Trans John Hull 1801 Sowler and Russell, Manchester, 101. In Colin Francombe *et al* 1993 *Caesarean Birth in Britain*. Middlesex University Press, London, 20.

[144] Colin Francombe *et al* 1993 op cit, 19.

[145] William Dease 1783 *Observations on Midwifery particularly on the Different Methods of Assisting Women in tedious and difficult Labours*. Williams White Wilson Byrne and Cash, Dublin, 61. In Jo Murphy- Lawless 1998 *Reading Birth and Death A History of Obstetric Thinking*. Cork University Press, Cork, 98.

[146] Ibid, 71. In ibid, 99.

also damned the procedure.[147] After looking at the evidence, he concluded that 'in no case whatever' should symphysiotomy be performed. It remained a marginal practice, used as a desperate measure, generally in Roman Catholic countries. The trial and error continued, however. A related operation, pubiotomy, that severed the pubic bone rather than the symphysis joint, was piloted in Naples in 1832.[148] The victim died the following night.

### A preference for craniotomy

Other solutions were available to the problem of obstructed labour before Caesarean section established itself as sufficiently safe to be an acceptable operation for general use. Doctors and midwives used a variety of techniques to turn the baby in those rare cases where the infant was presenting abnormally. Forceps operations were frequently used and the variety of obstetric forceps in use was wide. Where the infant had died, or where the mother could not be delivered by any other means, birth attendants resorted to craniotomy, an operation of last resort that crushed the baby's head in the womb. A related operation, embryotomy, where the infant's body was dismembered before being extracted was also practiced *in extremis*. These destructive operations — fatal to a child still living — appear to have been performed[149] in Europe and the United States in preference to symphysiotomy and pubiotomy in a pre-Caesarean era. Craniotomy was practised in Britain, it has been suggested, because British doctors privileged the life of the mother over that of the fetus. Medical policy in Britain favoured craniotomy in 1855, because it had a lower maternal death rate than Caesarean section.[150] The same obstetric policy held sway in Ireland. Irish doctors belonged to the same Royal College of Obstetricians and Gynaecologists in London as their British colleagues and professional ties between both countries were extremely strong.

---

[147] Alexander Hamilton 1803 *Outlines of the Theory and Practice of Midwifery*. 5th ed. T Kay, Edinburgh, 333. In Colin Francombe *et al* 1993 op cit, 19.

[148] Kenneth Bjorklund 2002 op cit.

[149] Edward Shorter 1983 *A History of Women's Bodies*. Allen Lane, London, 81-8.

[150] Colin Francombe *et al* 1993 op cit, 25.

## A revolution in Caesarean section

A German doctor, Max Sanger, revolutionised Caesarean section in 1882,[151] by developing a superior method of suturing the womb. Until then, doctors had been slow to stitch the uterus.[152] Obstetricians in both Britain and the United States debated the pros and cons of Caesarean section versus craniotomy. Tellingly, neither symphysiotomy nor pubiotomy featured in these professional disputes. At the annual general meeting of the British Medical Association in 1886, the contest was between Caesarean section and craniotomy.[153] Thirteen years later, the New York State Medical Association proposed that 'craniotomy should be abolished as a murderous procedure and Caesarian section substituted.'[154] By the end of the 19th century in Britain and the United States, Caesarean was beginning to be accepted as the treatment of choice for obstructed labour. By the early 1920s, Caesarean section had become popular in Britain.[155] While afficionados continued to sunder the joint of the *symphysis pubis*, 'symphysiotomy remained on the margins of mainstream obstetrics.'[156] Enthusiasm for pubiotomy was re-kindled briefly, however, by the invention in 1899 in Italy[157] of a modified chain saw for slicing through the pubic bone. Fourteen years after Gigli fashioned his twisted and barbed wire saw,[158] the operation of pubiotomy surfaced in Dublin, in the Coombe and Rotunda Hospitals. Dr Tweedy, the Rotunda's Master, considered pubiotomy preferable to craniotomy. In his 1907 report, he wrote that the 'new' operation had been performed five times.[159] The first patient to have her pubic bone sawn haemorrhaged from her genital lacerations, however, and was unable to walk for 63 days.

[151] Ibid, 32.
[152] M C O'Brien 1900 *Transactions of the New York State Medical Association for the year 1899* Vol (xvi): 88.
[153] Colin Francombe *et al* 1993 op cit, 33-4.
[154] M C O'Brien 1900 op cit.
[155] Colin Francombe *et al* 1993 op cit, 40.
[156] Janette Allotey 2007 *Discourses on the function of the pelvis from Ancient Times until the present day.* Unpublished Ph.D. thesis University of Sheffield.
[157] Kenneth Bjorklund 2002 op cit.
[158] Mark Skippen et al 2004 'The Chain Saw – A Scottish Invention.' *Scottish Medical Journal* 49 (2): 57-60.
[159] E H Tweedy 1908 'Clinical Reports of the Rotunda Hospital Dublin' *Journal of Medical Science* July-Dec cxxxv: 103. In Jo Murphy-Lawless 1998 op cit, 100.

Doctors in mainland Europe abandoned pubiotomy following the publication of an influential German article that revealed high numbers of women dying from its genital wounds.[160] Schafli's 1909 review of 672 pubiotomies showed that 32 women had died and that trauma to the sexual organs was the cause of death in 13 of these cases.[161] Enthusiasm for the surgery persisted at the Rotunda Hospital, however. Tweedy's successor, Jellett, was keen on the operation, particularly where disproportion was suspected during pregnancy,[162] and pubiotomy was performed at the Rotunda for a brief period from 1912-13. However, it is unlikely that either Tweedy or Jellett read German. Nor would they have had access to English language research on the surgery, as pubiotomy was no longer seen as acceptable practice among English-speaking obstetricians. Meanwhile, in Germany, doctors devised a subcutaneous form of the operation that was adopted in Argentina, a Catholic country. Dr Enrique Zarate of Buenos Aires advised 'only partial division of the symphysis with the knife, which is then completed by forceful abduction of the [mother's] thighs.'[163] His barbarous method later became popular at the Lourdes Hospital, although South African doctors[164] maintained that, without the modifications they themselves advised, Zarate's technique carried particular dangers.

---

160 Kenneth Bjorklund 2002 op cit.
161 A Schafli 1909. '700 Hebosteotomien.' *Z Geburtshilfe Gynakol* 64: 85 – 135.
162 Jo Murphy Lawless 1998 op cit, 100.
163 D Maharaj and J Moodley 2002 'Symphysiotomy and fetal destructive operations.' *Best Practice and Research Clinical Obstetrics and Gynaecology* 16 (1) : 117-131.
164 Crichton D and Seedat EK 1963 'The technique of symphysiotomy.' *South African Medical Journal* 37: 227-31.

# V 'Ireland stands alone': the revival of symphyiotomy

*Ireland stands alone in her fight to defend the Judeo-Christian moral code of sexual behaviour and the sanctity of life.*

Professor Emeritus John Bonnar,
addressing the Knights of Columbanus *circa* 1981.[165]

## Women and society

The Ireland of the 1940s has famously been described as 'a living tomb for women'.[166] De Valera's 1937 Constitution had positioned women as the bearers of children and the makers of bread. Female emigration was high, women faced government restrictions in employment and few married women worked outside the home. For many families, it was a time of poverty, but not of malnutrition. Rickets, for example, was rare.[167]

Looked at from a wider social perspective, these were dark decades. Religious and social prejudices against contraceptive use were widespread, and infanticide was still prevalent. Pregnancy outside marriage was harshly punished, with women dispatched to county homes, mother and baby homes and Magdalen laundries. Backstreet abortions were vigorously prosecuted by the authorities, and venereal disease was rife.[168] Cases of sexual abuse were frequently before the courts, although perpetrators were not often convicted.[169] Thousands

---

[165] Diarmaid Ferriter 2009 *Occasions of Sin: Sex and Society in Modern Ireland.* Profile, London, 470.

[166] Nuala O Faoláin 1996 *Are You Somebody? The Accidental Memoir of a Dublin Woman.* Henry Holt and Company, New York, 15.

[167] W J E Jessop 1950 *The Irish National Nutrition 1950 Survey Conference Proceedings.* Vol IV The Stationary Office, Dublin, 289-92.

[168] Diarmaid Ferriter 2009, 267.

[169] Diarmaid Ferriter 2009 op cit, 245.

of children were committed to 'orphanages' and to industrial and reform schools.

---

**8. Myths and red herrings**

'Everyone accepted ' authority' – especially that of the Church. Family sizes were very large and any woman starting her reproductive career at a young age could expect to have many further pregnancies'. Conor Carr, former Chairman of the Institute of Obstetricians and Gynaecologists, 2010.[170]

---

**Family planning**

The decline in family size in Ireland began a hundred years ago. From 1911-46, families shrank by 20 per cent.[171] There was some evidence of a trade in contraceptives in Dublin in 1929, with a small number of chemists and other outlets selling goods[172] whose importation was against the law. Section 17 of the 1935 Criminal Law (Amendment) Act prohibited the sale and importation of birth control devices. By then however, information on birth control was circulating among the middle classes.[173]

The Second World War intensified changes in sexual behaviour. Attitudes towards contraception were also influenced by fears of a global 'population bomb'. By the early 1950s, British newspapers and magazines, some containing articles on family planning, were flooding into Ireland.[174] While the 1929 Censorship Act explicitly prohibited publications advocating contraception, the banning of periodicals was outside the board's powers.[175] By the 1950s, limiting one's family was no

---

[170] Conor Carr 2010 'Symphysiotomy helped women have multiple births'. Letter *Irish Medical Times* 25 March.
[171] Diarmaid Ferriter 2009 op cit, 297.
[172] Ibid, 194.
[173] Ibid, 195.
[174] Michael Solomons 1992 *Pro Life? The Irish Question*. Lilliput Press, Dublin, 7.
[175] Diarmaid Ferriter 2009 op cit, 305.

longer sinful, according to the Catholic Church. While prohibiting artifical methods of contraception, the Church did not condemn birth control in principle. Addressing Catholic midwives in 1951, Pius XII justified the use of the 'safe period'[176] This moment marked a crucial shift in attitude, acording to Holles St historian Tony Farmar: 'once the Church declared that deliberately limiting one's family was in itself not sinful, it increasingly seemed to ordinary Catholics that the argument over the techniques used (short of abortion) was more technical than substantial.'

Statistical evidence suggests a degree of family planning in Dublin in the mid-1940s.[177] Women classified as 'professional and commercial' accounted for one in every 20 first babies born during the period 1943-45, but only one in every 200 eighth child or higher: two thirds of such infants were born to mothers married to unskilled workers. In 1946, just 38 per cent of children lived in families of five dependent children or more. Irish couples married for 30-34 years had on average 3.94 children on average.[178] By the end of the 1940s, notwithstanding the teaching of the Catholic Church on the issue, 'the mutilating operation of sterilisation' seemed to be well established, as Dr Alex Spain, Master of NMH and revivalist of symphysiotomy, noted with repugnance.[179]

This increasing 'laxity' on the part of Catholic women formed part of the background to the infamous battle between Church and State over the Mother and Child scheme. The Church opposed free maternity care for lower income mothers, seeing the scheme as a threat to the future of Catholic hospitals and a hazard to the morals of Catholic mothers. State medical officers could not be trusted to instruct Catholic girls and women in 'sex relations, chastity and marriage' according to Catholic principles. In a letter to Minister for Health Noel Browne in 1950, the Bishops also noted that 'gynaecological care' in some

---

[176] Tony Farmar 1994 *Holles Street 1894-1994 The National Maternity Hospital–A Centenary History.* Farmar, Dublin, 152.

[177] Tony Farmar 1994 op cit, 116.

[178] Diarmaid Ferriter 2009 op cit, 297.

[179] Alex Spain 1949 'Symphysiotomy and pubiotomy. An apologia based on the study of 41 cases'. *Journal of Obstetrics and Gynaecology of the British Empire* 56: 576-85.

countries was 'interpreted to include provision for birth limitation and abortion.'[180] The scheme was defeated in 1951 through the combined might of the Catholic Church and the medical profession. John Charles McQuaid, the Archbishop of Dublin, led on the side of the Church. His *porte parole*, one of two within the Irish Medical Association, was Dr John Cunningham, a consultant obstetrician at the National Maternity Hospital and its Master from 1931-41.[181]

The downward trend in family size continued: couples marrying in the 1950s continued to have fewer children.[182] In 1954, just 23 per cent of Irish couples had five children or more.[183] By then, Dr Arthur Barry, Master of NMH, was complaining that obstetricians — in his hospital, presumably — were under pressure to perform a hysterectomy following Caesarean section.[184] Dublin demographics in 1955 showed that fewer women were having a sixth child, or more, compared with a decade previously, and this was true of all social groups.[185] Just 8 per cent of all Dublin mothers were giving birth to a fifth baby: nationally, the figure was 9.8 per cent. Social class differences were sharp: the average number of previous children born to 'wage earners' was double that born to 'higher professionals'. There was also a trend towards older motherhood among higher income women.

### Holles St Hospital
Holles St Hospital was founded to provide a Catholic maternity facility for a largely Catholic population. Its chaplain, the Archbishop of Dublin, was seen as the ultimate authority on all hospital matters. He was also Chairman of the Board of Governors and parish priest of St Andrew's, the hospital's parish.[186] John Charles McQuaid controlled all

---

[180] John Cooney 1999 *John Charles McQuaid Ruler of Catholic Ireland.* O'Brien Press, Dublin, 258-9.

[181] Ibid, 298-305.

[182] Diarmaid Ferriter 2009 op cit, 297.

[183] Ibid, 301.

[184] Arthur Barry 1954 'Conservatism in Obstetrics'. *Transactions of the 6th International Congress of Catholic Doctors* John Fleetwood Ed. Guild of St Luke, SS Cosmas and Damian, Dublin, 122-6. In Jacqueline K Morrissey 2004 op cit, 155.

[185] J F Knaggs 1958 '*Natality in Dublin in the Year 1955*.' Address to the Statistical and Social Inquiry of Ireland 17 Jan.

[186] Tony Farmar 1994 op cit, 154.

hospital appointments[187] and took a keen interest in medical matters, keeping a particularly watchful eye on developments in obstetrics and gynaeology. 'Birth-prevention', in his view, was a 'crime'.[188]

---

### 9. Myths and red herrings

'In these years [1940s and 1950s] sepsis was one of the leading causes of maternal death. From 1950 onwards, the operation of symphysiotomy for obstructed labour was gradually replaced by the modern cesearean [sic] section; by then antibiotics were available to treat infection and sepsis became much less of a hazard.' John Bonnar, Chairman of the Institute of Obstetricians and Gynaecologists, 2001.[189]

---

### Caesarean section

While the Rotunda performed the first institutional Caesarean in Ireland in 1889,[190] it took several decades for the operation to become popular. By the end of the 1930s, however, Caesarean section had become the norm for difficult births in Ireland. By then, the spectre of maternal death had receded. Maternal mortality was no longer the main concern of obstetricians in the 1940s and 1950s, as alleged.[191] Deaths from puerperal fever, a common cause of maternal mortality for many years, had declined dramatically. Maternal mortality from Caesarean had fallen significantly. Surgical technique improved, blood transfusions became available, and aseptic and antiseptic drills were introduced: all helped to make the surgery safer. The advent of new drugs, such as sulphonamides, was also seen as critical to combating infection, although deaths from sepsis had receded before such medication came on stream. Maternal mortality almost halved at Holles St between 1935-40, halving again during the period 1940-45. By 1946, the rate at which women were dying in childbirth had fallen to

---

[187] John Cooney 1999 op cit, 340.
[188] Ibid, 277.
[189] John Bonnar 2001 Letter to Dr Jim Kiely, Chief Medical Officer, Department of Health and Children. 4 May.
[190] Jo Murphy-Lawless 1998 op cit, 99.
[191] Peter Boylan and Tony Farmar 1999 op cit.

1.20 per 1,000, while the rate for Ireland as a whole was 2.39 per 1,000,[192] half of what it had been in 1931.[193]

But however relatively safe it may have been, medically, Caesarean section could be seen to harbour other risks. The operation had been associated with sterilisation since the time of Porro in 1876, whose technique entailed removing the uterus to reduce the risks of haemhorrhage and infection.[194] While the Porro operation became obsolete, sterilisation following Caesarean section continued to be common practice. Figures published in Britain in 1920 suggested that two patients in every five had been sterilised in this way.[195]

---

### 10. Myths and red herrings

'It was not infrequent for the woman with the contracted pelvis to become pregnant again. If she had had a Caesarean section, there was a significant risk of a ruptured uterus. This was a very serious problem.' John R McCarthy, 2010.[196]

---

Doctors adopted a policy of repeat Caesareans, fearing to allow vaginal birth following Caesarean. A 1922 editorial in the British medical press complained about the 'mad rage for Caesarean section', saying it was being abused by being performed for varicose veins and epilepsy.[197] The editorial writer cautioned that, in a classic Caesarean, there was a risk the scar might rupture in a subsequent pregnancy, and suggested that the newer 'lower segment' operation would diminish this danger. (The classic Caesarean was a vertical cut into the uterus: the lower segment incision, being horizontal as well as lower, was less disruptive, less vulnerable to rupture and therefore safer.) British doctors, like their American counterparts, moved away from

---

[192] Tony Farmar 1994 op cit, 114.

[193] J.C. Saunders 1933 'Ireland: Maternal Mortality in Cork'. *British Medical Journal* 4 March 1(3765): 386-7.

[194] Colin Francombe *et al* 1993 op cit, 31.

[195] Ibid, 38-9.

[196] John R McCarthy 2010 'Controversy over childbirth operation'. Letter *The Irish Times* 1 March.

[197] *British Medical Journal* 1922: 277-8. In Colin Francombe *et al* 1993 op cit, 40.

a rigid policy of 'once a Caesarean, always a Caesarean' permitting vaginal birth after Caesarean in selected cases.[198] As an authoritative American text explained: 'most women after one cesarean [sic], especially it if was of the cervical [lower segment] kind, can go through pregnancy and labor safely again.'[199] This was the practice at NMH, where, in 1949, as many as 25 women gave birth vaginally following a previous Caesarean section for disproportion.[200]

The policy of repeat Caesareans, where followed, brought its own hazards, as good practice was generally seen to limit the number of Caesareans that could safely be performed. A 1931 English text by a former Assistant Master at the Rotunda proposed a solution: tubal ligation. 'If the [Caesarean section] patient has had previous operations, the question of sterilisation will arise, and each case must be decided on its merits'[201] But this was not a solution that Irish doctors were prepared to adopt. Hysterectomy, a more invasive operation that could more easily be cloaked under 'medical necessity', was preferred by those obstetricians who were prepared to accede to their patients' demands.[202] Tubal ligation, although legal in Ireland, was almost unobtainable: obstetricians refused to perform it for religious reasons.[203]

There was disagreement as to how many Caesarean sections a woman could safely undergo. Dr Alex Spain, for example, asserted that the dangers of repeat Caesarean were exaggerated. He argued strongly for the safety of the lower segment Caesarean, a view that was widely shared by his colleagues. The Master claimed that he himself had performed this lower segment operation seven times upon the same

---

[198] Colin Francombe *et al* 1993 op cit, 39.
[199] M Edward Davis and Mabel  C Cameron 1945 *DeLee's Obstetrics For Nurses* Saunders, Philadelphia.
[200] Jacqueline K Morrisey 2004 An examination of the relationship between the Catholic Church and the medical profession in Ireland in the period 1922 – 1992, with particular emphasis on the impact of this relationship in the field of reproductive medicine. Unpublished PhD thesis University College Dublin,162.
[201] Richard E Tottenham 1931 *A Handbook of Midwifery.* Churchill, London, 242.
[202] Maureen Harding Clark 2006 *The Lourdes Hospital Inquiry. An Inquiry into peripartum hysterectomy at Our Lady of Lourdes Hospital Drogheda Report of Judge Maureen Harding Clark SC* Jan. The Stationary Office, Dublin, 96.
[203] Jacqueline K Morrissey 2004 op cit, 183.

patient, to no ill-effect.[204] No upper limit, in his view, should be set to the number of such repeat Caesareans.

One of the main risks of repeat Caesareans was that the womb might rupture, but while this was an extremely serious complication, it very seldom happened. An authoritative London text put the overall risk of a ruptured uterus during labour at 1 in 6,000 in 1947.[205] This was borne out by statistics from the main Dublin maternity hospitals from 1940-50, which showed an incidence of (fatal) cases of 1.6 per 100,000,[206] but the data did not distinguish between classic and lower segment Caesarean.[207] However, the case for symphysiotomy was not made by revivalists on the basis that women were less at risk of dying from symphysiotomy than from Caesarean.

### Reviving symphysiotomy

Effectively a specialty of tropical obstetrics in other countries, symphysiotomy and pubiotomy were revived in Ireland in the 1940s. While the surgery is widely believed to have been exhumed at the National Maternity by Dr Alex Spain in 1944, symphysiotomy has been reported at St Finbarr's Hospital, Cork, as early as 1941.[208] Spain succeeded Dr John Cunningham — an *afficionado* of symphysiotomy and close *confidante* of John Charles McQuaid — as Master of Holles St Hospital in 1942. Conditions there were poor. So overcrowded was the hospital that local women were being implored to have their babies at home, while inpatients were being discharged early.[209] Symphysiotomy offered an alternative to Caesarean section that needed neither theatre nor electricity. All the ten-minute surgery required was a scalpel, a pair of surgical gloves, a local anaesthetic and a urinary catheter.[210]

---

[204] Alex Spain 1944 'National Maternity Hospital Report 1944' *Irish Journal of Medical Science* 1945: 474. In Jacqueline K Morrissey 2004 op cit, 154.

[205] Wilfred Shaw 1947 *A Textbook of Midwifery.* 2nd ed. Churchill, London, 438.

[206] Tony Farmar 1994 op cit, 121.

[207] Jacqueline K Morrissey 2004 op cit, 178.

[208] Sean Hurley 2003 Letter to Jan O'Sullivan TD 11 July.

[209] Tony Farmar 1994 op cit, 117-9.

[210] Kenneth Bjorklund 2002 'Minimally invasive surgery for obstructed labour: a review of symphysiotomy during the twentieth century (including 5000 cases)'. *British Journal of Obstetrics and Gynaecology* 109 (3): 236-48.

Symphysiotomy and pubiotomy had been shunned for many decades due to 'their many complications: haemorrhage, urinary fistulas, walking troubles.'[211] Spain was well aware of the opprobrium attaching to the surgery in the English-speaking world. The norm for obstructed labour, as he well knew, was Caesarean section.[212] Most mainstream English texts in obstetrics from the mid-18th century to the mid-20th century contained chapters on the deformed pelvis and the use of forceps, relegating symphysiotomy and pubiotomy to the margins of obsolescence.[213] If they were tolerated at all, it was only as operations of last resort. One classic 1947 text[214] dismissed them as 'obsolete, even with emergency cases [of contracted pelvis].'

Contrary to what the IOG has claimed, symphysiotomy and pubiotomy were not often performed as emergency procedures in Dublin in the 1940s and 50s. Historian Jacqueline Morrissey has rightly drawn attention to the fact that NMH obstetricians set out to revive the surgery as an elective or non-emergency procedure.[215] They were strongly criticised for doing so by a number of eminent British obstetricians, including Professor A S Duncan of the University of Wales.[216]

The advent of x-rays in Holles St in 1937[217] had boosted pelvimetry, the measurement of the pelvis, which had been done manually since the 18th century. Doctors saw women as inadequate, even to give birth: they felt 'a need to rescue women from their own bodies.'[218] Women's pelvises were widely believed to be the wrong size or the wrong shape and doctors suspected disproportion where it did not exist. If

---

[211] M Dumont 1989 'The long and difficult birth of symphysiotomy or from Severin Pineau to Jean-Rene Sigault' *Journal de Gynécologie, Obstétrique et Biologie de la Reproduction* 18(1):11-21.

[212] Alex Spain 1944 op cit. In Jacqueline K Morrissey 2004 op cit, 154.

[213] Janette Allotey 2007 *Discourses on the function of the pelvis from Ancient Times until the present day.* Unpublished Ph.D. thesis. University of Sheffield, 198.

[214] Wilfred Shaw 1947 *A Textbook of Midwifery.* 2nd ed. Churchill, London, 408.

[215] Jacqueline K Morrisey 2004 op cit, 153.

[216] Ibid, 167.

[217] Tony Farmar 1994 op cit, 107.

[218] Jo Murphy-Lawless 1998 op cit, 96.

inaccurate, pelvimetry could could lead to a misdiagnosis of disproportion, which in turn could herald a symphysiotomy. Some obstetricians were obsessed with pelvic measurements: pregnant women and their babies were routinely subjected to large doses of radiation, which was known to be toxic from the late 1950s. Disproportion was associated with a small or contracted pelvis. However, a contracted pelvis was very rare, and true disproportion was extremely uncommon. Nearly every woman was able to give birth to the child she bore, vaginally, as later research showed.[219]

---

**11. Myths and red herrings**

'The historic use of symphysiotomy should be assessed in the context of what was considered valid practice at the time. Medical research papers regarding symphysiotomy were produced from other countries at the time when the technique was being performed here.' Institute of Obstetricians and Gynaecologists, 2010.[220]

---

Symphysiotomy and pubiotomy were revived to deal with disproportion, where there was some lack of fit between the baby's head and its mother's pelvis: cases of gross disproportion, however, were to be treated by Caesarean section. The revival of the surgery at Holles St did not go unchallenged. The Royal Academy of Medicine, where the annual clinical reports of the main Dublin maternity hospitals were discussed, including by guest speakers from abroad, provided an arena for such challenges. Dr Bethel Solomons of the Rotunda was one of the first doctors to query the safety of symphysiotomy asking why NMH was reintroducing an operation that had been the subject of negative reports.[221] Like Dr Tweedy of the Rotunda 40 years earlier, Spain had little to guide his clinical practice

---

[219] Kieran O Driscoll, Declan Meagher with Peter Boylan 1993 *Active Management of Labor The Dublin Experience* 3rd ed. Mosby, London, 65.

[220] Institute of Obstetricians and Gynaecologists of the Royal College of Physicians of Ireland 2010 'Statement on Symphysiotomy' 17 Feb.

[221] *Royal Academy of Medicine in Ireland Transactions: Section of Obstetrics 1945. Irish Journal of Medical Science* 1946: 565. In Jacqueline K Morrissey op cit 2004, 159-60.

when he decided to revive these genitally wounding operations. The only reported accounts of symphysiotomy during the period 1900-44 were in German, Spanish and French.[222] Assuming Spain did not read such 'foreign' languages, there was little available to him by way of contemporaneous evidence, apart from a few decades-old case histories from the Rotunda. But whether or not he was operating in the dark, Spain used his considerable power as Master to drive symphysiotomy and pubiotomy in his hospital.

Writing in the hospital's annual report, Spain acknowledged the difficulty of performing an operation that was held in such low esteem by his colleagues: 'that I have not employed it more frequently is due to the fact that it was an entirely new procedure to me and one that has to be faced against the weight of opinion of the entire English speaking obstetrical world'.[223] Despite this, Spain persevered, and by the final year of his mastership, he had symphysiotomised 43 women.[224]

Spain's successor at NMH, Dr Arthur Barry was an even more fervent devotee of symphysiotomy and pubiotomy: the hospital performed 165 of these operations during his term as Master, from 1949-55.[225] Under his tutelage, the surgery spread to other Catholic teaching hospitals, such as the Coombe, where Master John Kevin Feeney rivalled Barry, carrying out 137 of these surgeries from 1950-56,[226] despite the Coombe's lower number of births. Addressing a medical congress in Dublin in 1954, Barry set out to persuade his colleagues to adopt symphysiotomy on the basis that it promoted 'natural' or or non-Caesarean birth in future pregnancies. After acknowledging the safety of Caesarean section, Barry argued that symphysiotomy or pubiotomy should be the 'obstetric procedure of choice' for 'minor to medium disproportion'. He rested his case on the need to preserve women's

---

[222] Kenneth Bjorklund 2002 op cit.

[223] *National Maternity Hospital Report 1948*: 456 *Irish Journal of Medical Science* 1949. in Jacqueline K Morrisey 2004 op cit, 158.

[224] Ibid.

[225] *National Maternity Hospital Report 1955 Irish Journal of Medical Science* 1956. In Jacqueline K Morrisey 2004 op cit, 159.

[226] *Coombe Lying-In Hospital Report 1956 Irish Journal of Medical Science* 1957. In Jacqueline K Morrisey 2004 op cit, 175-6.

reproductive capacity to the full: 'this relatively simple and minor procedure will give rise to a permanent and stable enlargement of the pelvis so that the individual will ... be able to have natural [or non-Caesarean] births whenever she desires'.[227]

While much was claimed for the surgery, hospital records showed high levels of fetal deaths and fetal injuries. Rotunda doctors criticised the practice, which they eschewed.[228] In 1951, Dr O'Donel Browne, Master of the Rotunda, pleaded with Holles St Hospital obstetricians to desist from symphysiotomy, pointing out that Caesarean section would result in less loss of life to mothers and babies and fewer injuries.[229] But the comparative research was never undertaken, as Dr Jacqueline Morrissey has underlined. No figures were ever produced by either NMH or the Coombe comparing the respective outcomes of symphysiotomy wth those of Caesarean section for either mothers or for babies.[230]

British obstetricians of the time, notably Professor Jeffcoate of Liverpool University, were horrified by the number of fetal deaths from symphysiotomy at NMH and by the babies born so starved of oxygen that they were likely to have been brain damaged. He punctured Barry's grandiose claim for symphysiotomy and pubiotomy ('what we offer is a *cure* for disproportion, not a treatment which has to be repeated with each pregnancy'[231]) by pointing to six cases of symphysiotomy where the baby had to be delivered by forceps, and one where the mother needed to be delivered by Caesarean section. In many of these births, he said, the babies were already distressed by the time of the operation, and Caesarean would have offered them certain and immediate relief. Jeffcoate underlined that one baby born by symphysiotomy had died,

---

227 Arthur Barry 1954 'Conservatism in Obstetrics'. *Transactions of the 6<sup>th</sup> International Congress of Catholic Doctors* John Fleetwood ed. Guild of St Luke, SS Cosmas and Damian, Dublin, 122-6.
228 Jacqueline K Morrisey 2004 op cit, 162.
229 *Royal Academy of Medicine in Ireland Transactions: Section of Obstetrics 1951. Irish Journal of Medical Science* 1951: 1031. In ibid, 166-7.
230 Ibid, 187.
231 *Royal Academy of Medicine in Ireland Transactions: Section of Obstetrics 1950. Irish Journal of Medical Science* 1950: 866. In ibid, 159.

while several others had been born 'in a state of severe asphyxia'. Time would tell ' whether they sustained asphyxial necrosis [tissue death] of the brain cortex [stem]'.[232] Barry later attempted to counter Jeffcoate's criticisms by asserting that the operation had been proven to overcome disproportion, that it was safe, and that NMH had not encountered any significant risks or long term complications.[233]

His claim that symphysiotomy offered a permanent remedy for disproportion was belied by the number of instances where symphysiotomy was followed by Caesarean section, either in the birth in hand or in a subsequent pregnancy. Cases where symphysiotomy was carried out on women who had previously undergone a Caesarean and where the baby had to be delivered by repeat Caesarean notwithstanding the pelvis-sundering procedure[234] also highlighted the futility of the surgery.

Professor Chassar Moir of Oxford University was as appalled as Jeffcoate at the revival of the surgery at NMH and roundly attacked symphysiotomy as a procedure that killed infants: 'Is it then your policy to sacrifice the firstborn baby and to use its dead or dying body as nothing more than a battering ram to stretch its mother's pelvis in the hope that subsequent brothers and sisters may thereby have (possibly) an easier entrance into this world?' he asked.

Chassar Moir also underlined the superiority of Caesarean section from the mother's perspective, saying that 'a woman who has been many hours in heavy labour makes a quicker and better recovery after abdominal delivery'.[235] But the surgery, which was almost as risky for mothers as it was for babies, was rarely considered from the woman's point of view. Its Dublin promoters were seemingly unaware of papers from Spain — the only other country in the Western world where sporadic outbreaks of symphysiotomy were recorded — testifying to

---

[232] Ibid, 861. In ibid, 161-2.

[233] Ibid,163.

[234] Ibid, 172.

[235] *Royal Academy of Medicine in Ireland Transactions: Section of Obstetrics* 1951. *Irish Journal of Medical Science* 1951: 1026. In ibid, 164.

the operation's relatively high death rate for mothers compared with Caesarean section. [236]

Little or no attempt was made in Dublin to calculate the cost to the mother of these genitally wounding procedures. Failure to locate the joint of the symphysis pubis, for example, was one of the known complications of symphysiotomy.[237] Doctors resolved this difficulty by performing a pubiotomy, where the bone was cut instead of the joint, resulting in a compound fracture of the pelvis, according to a 1931 text.[238] Professor Ian Donald of Glasgow University compared the skeletal damage inflicted by symphysiotomy with the less injurious (he implied) soft tissue injury from Caesarean. He expressed concern about the possibility that the operation would result in stress incontinence in later life.[239] Professor A Davidson expressed disbelief in the data published by NMH on these operations, particularly in relation to the apparent absence of walking difficulties and urinary troubles.[240] Once again, assertion took the place of evidence. Dr Feeney of the Coombe also asserted the operation's safety, saying that there were no long-term consequences — as far as doctors knew.[241] However, patients were not followed over time to determine the long-term consequences, and apart from a mere 18 cases, no longitudinal research was ever done in Dublin to establish the surgery's long-term side effects for mothers.[242]

Symphysiotomy's high death rate for babies was later acknowledged both by Barry and by Feeney. 'The real harvest of symphysiotomy is reaped in subsequent deliveries,'[243] Feeney wrote. He later

[236] S Dexeus and N Salarich 1954. 'De la sinfisiotomia complementaria de recurso o de emergencia en el curso de la extraccion fetal por las vias naturales'. *Revista Espagnola de Obstetricia y Ginecologia* 13:358 – 366.
[237] Jacqueline K Morrissey 2004 op cit, 177.
[238] Richard E Tottenham 1931 *A Handbook of Midwifery*. Churchill, London, 242.
[239] *Royal Academy of Medicine in Ireland Transactions: Section of Obstetrics* 1955. *Irish Journal of Medical Science* 1955: 530. In Jacqueline K Morrissey 2004 op cit, 168.
[240] *Royal Academy of Medicine in Ireland Transactions: Section of Obstetrics* 1956. *Irish Journal of Medical Science* 1956: 526. In Jacqueline K Morrissey 2004 op cit, 168.
[241] *Coombe Lying-In Hospital Report 1956* op cit, 1949-50. In ibid, 176.
[242] Ibid, 187.
[243] *Coombe Lying-In Hospital Report 1954 Irish Journal of Medical Science* 1955: 51. In ibid, 186.

acknowledged that symphysiotomy carried a 10 per cent mortality rate for babies,[244] while Barry attributed just 12 infant deaths directly to the surgery in 165 NMH cases.[245] In all, 19 babies died in these symphysiotomies and pubiotomies, however. Barry had previously published a selective account of 42 operations in the medical press[246] that omitted 11 other cases performed in the same time period, including four where the baby was stillborn. One of these cases was a pubiotomy — done after doctors had failed to identify the *symphysis pubis* joint — that was wrongly classified as a symphysiotomy in the hospital report. [247]

**The Africa connection**
The shadow of Africa loomed large over the 'new' surgery. One of Spain's objectives was to develop NMH as an international centre for training in obstetrics and gynaecology. Symphysiotomy was pivotal to this ambition: the theatreless operation was seen to be 'enormously useful as a substitute for Caesarian (sic) section in conditions in Africa and India where major surgery was not possible'.[248] Also, certain African cultures were believed to have a cultural bias against abdominal delivery (Caesarean section).

Future Medical Missionaries of Mary had trained in Holles St since 1936, before the order was founded.[249] They went to Nigeria the following year. By 1944, the year of symphysiotomy's revival, the nuns' hospital at Anua, Nigeria, was well established. Two years later, three sister clinics were up and running, including one in Afikpo,[250] which was later to become an important centre of symphysiotomy.[251]

---

[244] *Coombe Lying-In Hospital Report 1956* op cit, 1949-50. In ibid, 175.
[245] Ibid, 173.
[246] Arthur Barry 1952 'Symphysiotomy Why? When? How?' *Irish Journal of Medical Science* (Feb) 121: 49-73. In Jacqueline K Morrissey op cit 2004.
[247] In ibid, 177-8.
[248] Tony Farmar 1994 op cit, 114.
[249] See: http://medicalmissionariesofmary.com/index.php/mmm-milestones/216-an-extraordinary-adventure
[250] Ibid.
[251] IM Sunday-Adeoye, P Okonta and D Twomey 2004 'Symphysiotomy at the Mater Misericordiae Hospital Afikpo, Ebonyi State of Nigeria (1982-1999): a review of 1013 cases'. *Journal of Obstetrics and Gynaecology* Jan 24 (5): 525-529.

## The Catholic rule

NMH obstetricians ignored the pleas from Dr O'Donel Browne, Master of the Rotunda, to desist from the practice of symphysiotomy. Holles St stood firm. Symphysiotomy was a moral issue.[252] As Professor John Cunningham, McQuaid's man in the Irish Medical Association during the Mother and Child negotiations[253] and a consultant obstetrican at NMH, later wrote: 'in Roman Catholic countries, efforts to perfect the operation [of symphysiotomy] have been sustained. Contraception and sterilisation are not countenanced by those who subscribe to the Catholic rule.'[254] The medical profession had been opposed to artificial contraception since the 1880s, when contraceptive devices were first marketed in Britain.[255] Birth control not only conflicted with social mores, it was associated with classes of persons not considered respectable and was additionally seen to represent a threat to medical authority and professional status. Moreover, Catholic doctors, such as Cunningham and Spain, opposed Caesarean section on ethical grounds, seeing it as facilitating sterilisation and encouraging contraception, both practices that were prohibited by the Catholic Church.

Free-thinking, post-war Britain posed a threat to traditional Catholic values in Ireland. Spain argued against Caesarean section on moral grounds even in the medical press, saying that, if doctors perform it, 'the results will be contraception, the mutilating operation of sterilisation, and marital difficulty'. These were matters 'of immense importance in any community, especially where the great body or any large number of the people subscribe to the Catholic rule'. The obstetrician, he believed, was required to take the long view: 'such a solution [Caesarean section], although it will often get one out of immediate difficulty is not a long term answer; and this is the kernel of

---

[252] Jacqueline K Morrissey op cit 2004, 185.
[253] John Cooney 1999 *John Charles McQuaid Ruler of Catholic Ireland.* O'Brien Press, Dublin, 298-305.
[254] John Cunningham 1959. In Eardley Holland and Aleck Bourne Eds *British Obstetric and Gynaecological Practice.* 2nd ed. Heinemann, London.
[255] John S Haller and Robin M Haller 1974. *The Physician and Sexuality in Victoria America.* University of Illinois Press, Chicago.

the matter — the obstetrician must look to the future.'[256] As Arthur Barry later explained, taking the long view meant acting as the patient's moral guardian. 'The word obstetrician means the one who stands between the woman and harm, and yet he is the one who blasts the married life of countless women by performing a [Caesarean] section in the first pregnancy for disproportion. This is followed so frequently by artificial interference with conception, by induction of criminal abortion, by marked limitation of family, and finally by the removal of the capacity to reproduce by tubal ligation.'[257]

With Barry at the helm, NMH was seen as 'an institution imbued with the full rigour of Catholic moral doctrine.'[258] In addition to being a Knight of Columbanus, he was also a member of the Guild of Saints Luke, Cosmas and Damian, an association of Catholic doctors dedicated to putting Catholic teaching into clinical practice. Under the guidance of Pope Pius XI, the Guild became a warhead for an international movement, FIAMC (*Fédération Internationale des Associations de Medecins Catholiques*), the World Federation of Catholic Medical Associations. One of FIAMC's earliest international congresses was held in Ireland in 1954. The conference, which was likely brought to Dublin by Barry, aimed to bring a Catholic medical perspective to the population bomb, or 'demography and its medical incidence'. The gathering was addressed by Archbishop McQuaid, who advised his medical audience to close ranks against theories and practices that were 'but a cancellation of human nature.'[259]

The keynote speaker was Arthur Barry. He advocated symphysiotomy on non-medical grounds, putting forward arguments not usually found in his writings in the medical press. He stressed that 'it is unnecessary to stress to Catholic doctors that the practices of contraception,

---

[256] Alex Spain 1949 'Symphysiotomy and pubiotomy An apologia based on the study of 41 cases'. *Journal of Obstetrics and Gynaecology of the British Empire.* 56:576-85.

[257] Arthur Barry 1950 *Royal Academy of Medicine in Ireland Transactions: Section of Obstetrics. Discussion of Dublin Maternity Reports 1950. Irish Journal of Medical Science*: 865. In Jacqueline K Morrisey op cit 2004, 156-7.

[258] Tony Farmar 1994 op cit, 136.

[259] John Cooney 1999 *John Charles McQuaid Ruler of Catholic Ireland* O'Brien Press, Dublin, 307.

sterilisation and therapeutic abortion are contrary to the moral law. But what we must all guard against, and especially is this so in the teaching centres, is the unwarranted and unnecessary employment of Caesarean section'. The NMH Master continued: 'Every Catholic obstetrician should realise that the Caesarean operation is probably the chief cause for the practice by the profession of the unethical procedure of sterilisation and furthermore it is very frequently responsible for encouraging the laity in the improper prevention of pregnancy or in seeking its termination ... That the lower segment [Caesarean] operation is the most satisfactory and logical line of treatment in gross disproportion is not for a moment to be questioned, but in cases of minor or medium disproportion, the relatively simple procedure of symphysiotomy which allows of vaginal delivery for this and all subsequent pregnancies must surely be the obstetric procedure of choice.' In conclusion, Barry wrote that he was not advising the abolition of Caesarean section, but he urged Catholic doctors to 'abandon it in most cases of disproportion. I have carried out the operation of symphysiotomy in over 100 cases in the past five years and can assure you that all the bogies and pitfalls mentioned in the textbooks are sheer flights of imagination .... You can do it in safety in all cases of mild or moderate disproportion, you can relieve the disproportion permanently at no expense to mother and child and thus you can reduce the temptation to perform many of the unethical procedures which we all so resent.' 'If you must cut something, cut the symphysis', he concluded.[260]

Published in 1955, the conference proceedings carried a message of support from Pope Pius XII, signed by Archbishop Montini, (later Pope Paul VI). Leading Churchmen, such as the Papal Nuncio, Archbishop Gerald O'Hara, Cardinal John Dalton, and John Charles McQuaid paid tribute to the 'brilliant minds' of the Catholic doctors who worked for the Faith.[261] The Dublin publication carried a formal seal of

---

[260] Arthur Barry 1954 'Conservatism in Obstetrics'. *Transactions of the 6th International Congress of Catholic Doctors* John Fleetwood Ed. Guild of St Luke, SS Cosmas and Damian, Dublin, 122-6.

[261] John Cooney 2003 'Catholic Church did urge doctors to use symphysiotomy operation' *Irish Times* 9 Sept.

approval: the imprimatur of Archbishop John Charles McQuaid: 'Nihil Obstat Conor Martin. Imprimi Potest, Ioannes Carolus, Archiep. Dublinen, Hiberniae Primas.'[262]

Twenty years later, Dr Mary Henry, a vascular physician, presented a paper to the Institute of Obstetricians and Gynaecologists on 23 women, all mothers of large families, who had died from a pulmonary embolism from 1966-73. She appealed for tubal ligation for her current patients, all of whom had previously suffered from deep vein thrombosis. 'The only contraceptive available at the time was a high dose pill, which was described as a cycle regulator and which was totally unsuitable for such women,' she later told the Senate. Her plea fell on deaf ears. One member of the IOG offered a solution, however, and reminded Dr Henry that she surely knew 'a friendly gynaecologist who would carry out hysterectomies on these patients.'[263]

**The Lourdes Hospital**
The hospital owned by the Medical Missionaries of Mary in Drogheda was another epicentre of symphysiotomy. Just qualified as midwives, the nuns were invited to take over a maternity home in Drogheda in 1939. This was the nucleus of the teaching hospital that was to become central to the order's African project. The nuns' medical ambition to run hospitals was also a religious mission: one of their main aims was to train medical staff for missionary work in developing countries. Initial recognition for the hospital from training bodies, such as the Nursing Board, came as early as 1942. Following a fire that destroyed the old hospital, the nuns built their new International Missionary Training Hospital to train doctors, nurses and midwives for Africa.[264]

Links between NMH and the Lourdes Hospital were strong, with Holles St acting as trainer and mentor to the fledgling order whose

---

[262] John Cooney, personal communication.
[263] Mary Henry 2006 Seanad Debates Lourdes Hospital Inquiry: Statements Vol 1 No 74 Col 2012. 9 March.
[264] http://medicalmissionariesofmary.com/index.php/mmm-milestones/218-new-horizons.

growing network of clinics and hospitals in Africa must have been an invaluable source of trainees for NMH. By the time the new hospital opened in Drogheda in 1957, the order had expanded its operations not only in Nigeria, but into East Africa, Angola, the United States and Italy. Taiwan, Kenya's Turkana Desert, Malawi, Ethiopia and Brazil followed. Former NMH Master, John Cunningham, was a 'honorary' consultant at the Lourdes in the years following the Mother and Child debacle.[265] His successor, Arthur Barry, oversaw the maternity unit until 1964, when a second consultant obstetrician was appointed there, [266] a former Assistant Master at NMH who was also a devotee of symphysiotomy. Barry remained 'visiting' consultant at the Lourdes until 1972-73.

Both hospitals had a shared ethic and both were under the control of Catholic Archdioceses. The influence of Catholic teaching on medical practice was particularly in evidence at the Lourdes Hospital. The Medical Missionaries of Mary occupied almost all the key roles at the hospital and its maternity unit. Medical consultants were required to sign contracts agreeing to abide by Catholic ethics. These were largely concerned with the control of reproduction. The nuns encouraged natural methods of family planning: advice on artificial methods was forbidden.[267] 'Some reluctance' to perform a Caesarean section on a woman having her first baby was reported and three Caesareans was said to be the upper (safety) limit. Medical records carried entries noting that Caesarean section had been performed on an 'elderly patient' (in her early 30s), for example, or on a woman who had been 'married 10 years'.[268]

The practice of symphysiotomy at the Lourdes Hospital appears to have begun with the appointment of its 'foundation obstetrician', Dr Gerard Connolly. He worked in Africa, in Sierra Leone and in Nigeria, spending three years at the nuns' hospital in Anua from 1942-45

[265] Sheila Martin 2009 *Symphysiotomy at Our Lady of Lourdes.* Unpublished diploma thesis, 1.
[266] Maureen Harding Clark 2006 op cit, 59.
[267] Maureen Harding Clark 2006 op cit, 233.
[268] Sheila Martin 2006 op cit, 9.

before returning to Drogheda to run their maternity unit. Instead of the more usual membership of the Royal College of Obstetricians and Gynaecologists (RCOG), he possessed a Master's degree in the 'Art of Obstetrics', acquired solely by way of written examination.[269] Conditions at the hospital were impoverished for many years, with one small, pokey theatre separated by a flight of stairs from the labour ward. There was no lift.

Connolly, who was described as 'a gentleman' and 'deeply religious',[270] was reputed to be friendly with John Charles McQuaid, a fellow Cavan man. Both were members of the Knights of Columbanus, a powerful Catholic men's society whose chief spiritual mentor was the Archbishop. Organised Catholic lay organisations, such as the Knights, were to the forefront of Catholic Action, a lay movement in the first half of the last century that sought to assert Catholic values and Catholic power in the new State. One of the Knights' objectives was to secure 'adequate recognition for Catholic doctrine and practices in all phases of life, social, public, commercial and professional.'[271] Connolly's religious beliefs carried into the practice of obstetrics and were shared by his employers. Contraception was not permitted and female sterilisation by tubal ligation was not an option'.[272] He was strongly opposed to artificial birth control[273] and carried out symphysiotomy 'in the hope of avoiding Caesarean section.'

His predilection for symphysiotomy was an open secret. He told the Royal Academy of Medicine in 1966 that he was aware of his reputation as an 'addict': 'if we cannot deliver with the vacuum extractor and [oxytocin] drip [given to induce or accelerate labour] we divide the symphysis'.[274] Connolly did hundreds of symphysiotomies at the

[269] Maureen Harding Clark 2006 op cit, 162.
[270] ibid
[271] Maurice Curtis 2009. *The Splendid Cause. The Catholic Action Movement in Ireland in the Twentieth Century.* Original Writing and Greenmount, Dublin, 71.
[272] Maureen Harding Clark 2006 op cit,162.
[273] Ibid, 233.
[274] Gerard Connolly 1966 *Royal Academy of Medicine in Ireland Transactions: Section of Obstetrics The annual reports of the Rotunda, Coombe and National Maternity Hospitals for the year 1964.* 7 Jan.

Lourdes Hospital: staff believed, rightly or wrongly, that he had brought the operation back with him from Africa. As Judge Maureen Harding Clark commented: 'it was very likely that Dr Connolly's skills were appropriate to the training of medical personnel on African missions...' where there were few colleagues, limited blood supplies and 'preserving fertility was of paramount importance in African culture and thus caesarean sections were a last resort'.[275] Testimony from survivors supports the view that they were used as 'clinical material' or teaching aids at the Lourdes. The operation persisted there until 1984, two years after Connolly had retired.

Medical records compiled at the Lourdes were detailed and painstaking, sketching childbearing over a woman's lifetime, with births categorised according to whether or not they were the fruits of symphysiotomy or Caesarean section, or both. Tables on how many women had a vaginal birth following a symphysiotomy in a previous pregnancy or birth were standard.

---

[275] Maureen Harding Clark 2006 op cit, 162.

# VI 'Who was the Hippocratic Oath for?' In the eyes of the law

*'Who was the Hippocratic Oath for? It certainly was not for mothers!'*
Anne Lyons, survivor of symphysiotomy.

### The standard of care

Looked at through the eyes of the law, the conclusion that symphysiotomy and pubiotomy were unlawful seems inescapable. Doctors failed 'to conduct their practice in accordance with the conduct of a prudent and diligent doctor in the same circumstances.'[276] Neither symphysiotomy nor pubiotomy formed part of the standard of care that might reasonably be expected of a competent member of the specialty of obstetrics and gynaecology in the Western world in 1944. While there was some very limited tolerance within these islands of symphysiotomy as an operation of last resort, pubiotomy was almost universally considered to be completely outside the limits of acceptable medical practice. The use of a 'circular' saw reported by some survivors strongly suggests that pubiotomy, not symphysiotomy, was performed. Unlike the severing of the bone in pubiotomy, the cutting of the cartilage in symphysiotomy would not have required the use of a Gigli saw. NMH policy was to resort to pubiotomy — misleadingly described in hospital reports as 'symphysiotomy' — if doctors failed to find the *symphysis pubis* joint. This is also likely to have been the practice in other hospitals, particularly at the Lourdes Hospital, which was effectively a satellite of Holles St.

Pubiotomy was a barbarous procedure at best that, left without appropriate treatment following surgery, could result in a lop-sided pelvis. Where pubiotomy was performed because doctors were incapable of identifying the symphysis pubis — a relatively simple joint

---

[276] John Seymour 2000 *Childbirth and the Law*. Oxford University Press, Oxford, 34

to locate — the operation involved sawing blindly through the bone without the symphysis to guide the saw. The recklessness of such random sawing is self-evident.

---

**12. Myths and red herrings:**
'At that time, symphysiotomy was a simpler and safer practice than caesarean section (C/S), a technique that gradually replaced it during the 20th century when difficulties with the C/S procedure itself were overcome.' Institute of Obstetricians and Gynaecologists, 2010.[277]

---

Had Spain and his successors been charged with negligence, they would have found it difficult to defend themselves. Apart from Ireland, Franco's Spain was the only country where isolated outbreaks of these operations were reported in the 1940s and '50s.[278] By 1944, symphysiotomy and pubiotomy had long been shunned in the Western World. Symphysiotomy had been jettisoned in France, the country of its birth, by the end of the 1700s. Pubiotomy fared even worse. Following a brief flurry after the invention of the Gigli chainsaw in 1899, the operation was virtually abandoned. Even Dr Kenneth Bjorklund, the author of a positive review of symphysiotomy, approved of pubiotomy's demise.[279] Symphysiotomy and pubiotomy also fell out of favour in the United States around the turn of the last century. The last time a pubic bone was sawn through in New York's Sloane Hospital, for example, was in 1902, while the last cutting of the symphysis took place there in 1908.[280] These operations never succeeded in establishing themselves as mainstream practice in Western obstetrics, as a study of

---

[277] Institute of Obstetricians and Gynaecologists 2010 'Statement on Symphysiotomy'. 17 Feb.

[278] Kenneth Bjorklund 2002 'Minimally invasive surgery for obstructed labour: a review of symphysiotomy during the twentieth century (including 5000 cases)'. *British Journal of Obstetrics and Gynaecology* 109 (3): 236-48.

[279] Ibid.

[280] Edward Shorter 1982 *A History of Women's Bodies*. Allen Lane, London, 163.

English texts shows.[281] Other destructive operations, such as craniotomy and embryotomy, were practiced *in extremis* in these islands in preference to symphysiotomy and pubiotomy.

By 1944, symphysiotomy had become a specialty of tropical medicine, or 'jungle obstetrics', to quote one South African doctor.[282] The conditions that prevailed in medicine in the tropics, however, hardly provided an appropriate medico-legal context in which to determine the relative risks and benefits of the surgery for Irish women in the mid-1940s. Apart from a few Rotunda case histories on pubiotomy from the 1910s, the most recent English-language article available to Spain had reportedly been published some 36 years earlier, in 1908,[283] while the only other paper readily available to him was an account of five operations published in 1902.[284] Between the dated nature of the evidence and the low number of cases involved in these accounts (73), Spain's evidential base for re-introducing symphysiotomy and pubiotomy was extremely weak.

He failed in his duty of care to his patients: if he had access to 'foreign language' articles, then the reported dangers of symphysiotomy and pubiotomy should have deterred him from embarking on these operations, and if his only access to information about the surgery was via English language papers, then he should have been restrained by his lack of knowledge and by the near universal rejection of these procedures by his peers.

By the end of the 1930s, Caesarean section had become the accepted treatment in Ireland for difficult births. To deviate from that norm in the absence of medical necessity was to engage in malpractice and negligence. A 1947 text states baldly that symphysiotomy and pubiotomy are no longer performed if the facilities for Caesarean section are available. Its author, a former examiner of midwifery and

---

[281] Janette Allotey 2007 *Discourses on the function of the pelvis from Ancient Times until the present day.* Unpublished Ph.D. thesis, University of Sheffield, 198.

[282] V J Hartfield 1975. 'Late effects of symphysiotomy'. *Tropical Doctor* 5: 76-8.

[283] Zweifel 1908 Subcutaneous symphysiotomy and extra-peritoneal Caesarean section. *British Medical Journal* 2: 801-804.

[284] RC Buist RC 1902 Symphysiotomy in domestic and hospital practice. *Journal of Obstetrics and Gynaecology of the British Empire* 2:32-9.

gynaecology at the Universities of Oxford and Cambridge, emphasised that, of the two operations, pubiotomy was the safer.[285] While Dr Wilfred Shaw was almost alone in this view, it does indicate the depth of suspicion in which symphsyiotomy was held by leading medical authorities if the era. And, while the practice of symphysiotomy and pubiotomy became customary in certain hospitals, it was not acceptable. 'Negligence cannot be excused on the grounds that others practice the same kind of negligence.'[286]

Suggestions that symphysiotomy was performed as an emergency procedure have been shown to be without foundation. Many survivors have testified that theirs was a planned or non-emergency operation and this is borne out overwhelmingly by hospital reports. Apart from a very rare medical emergency, these operations were planned. They were not honest errors of clinical judgement, such as might be made by a competent professional acting with due care in a medical emergency. They were deliberate and wilful acts of surgery that ignored the medical consensus of the day, driven by personal belief systems, that met individual and institutional medical and religious needs.

Some symphsyiotomies were more negligent than others. The practice of Caesarean symphysiotomy was utterly egregious. Never before in the history of the surgery had the double procedure been recorded, to judge from Bjorklund's review.[287] The performance of a childbirth operation that broke the pelvis in the absence of a baby to be delivered was indefensible. While symphyiotomy was touted by Arthur Barry as offering a permanent cure for disproportion, this was wishful thinking. The idea of 'permanently enlarging the pelvis' suggests a degree of precision and therefore of predictability, but the outcome of the surgery was imprecise and unpredictable, as the degree to which the pelvis might open in future births could not be foretold.[288] These operations were performed to avert the possibility of Caesarean section, either for

---

[285]   Wilfred Shaw 1947 *A Textbook of Midwifery.* 2nd ed. Churchill, London, 595.
[286]   John Seymour 2000 op cit, 35.
[287]   Kenneth Bjorklund 2002 op cit.
[288]   Janette Allotey, personal communication.

a baby as yet unconceived, as in Caesarean symphysiotomy, or for a baby as yet unborn, as in symphysiotomy during pregnancy. However, every labour is an unpredictable dynamic process, babies come in different sizes, and their heads (usually their biggest parts) have the ability to change position during labour. Sometimes the soft skull bones, especially before a baby becomes post mature, can override during the birth process and this makes the head slightly smaller. The mother's position and skeletal suppleness may also help. So operations done for disproportion two, four or six weeks before the mother's due date, could not be justified, as the degree to which the baby's head would mould during labour could not be predicted, nor the opening of the birth canal.[289] Not even for the birth in hand could symphsyiotomy be relied upon to offer a solution to the problem of obstructed labour. Where symphysiotomy failed, the baby was delivered by Caesarean section, and the mother was left with an unhinged pelvis.

Also, leading clinicians have queried the appropriateness of performing a symphsyiotomy in cases where the baby was in an unusually difficult position. They say, for example, that in the case of a breech presentation where the pelvic capacity is likely to be inadequate, the case for Caesarean section was overwhelming.[290] Why put the mother through that agony, they ask, when there is a possibility that Caesarean will be needed to deliver the aftercoming head of the infant if it becomes trapped? The same observation was made in respect of a brow presentation — reported by one survivor — a position that makes birthing a baby impossible for the mother unless the head flexes. Requiring a mother with an unhinged pelvis to try to deliver such a baby was indefensible, say clinicians. Mothers whose babies presented as breeches, as faces and even as brows were commonly delivered by symphysiotomy at the Lourdes Hospital.

Post operative care appears to have been extraordinarily deficient, both in hospitals and in the community. The spontaneous rupture of the *symphyis pubis* during childbirth had been described in 1933.[291] The

---

[289] Ibid.

[290] Mavis Kirkham, personal communication.

[291] B F Boland 1933 'Rupture of the symphysis pubis articulation during delivery.' *Surgery, Gynecology and Obstetrics* 57:517-522.

surgical rupture of the joint induced by symphsyiotomy was not materially different. Historically, spontaneous rupture was treated with 'bed rest, usually in a lateral decubitus [lying down] position, analgesics, and the application of a pelvic binder'[292] Had orthopaedic surgeons been consulted, they would likely have mandated such therapy for a minimum of six weeks following surgery, along with close supervision and follow up. This would, in all probability, have ameliorated the surgery's side effects.[293] Instead, more often than not, the patient whose pelvis had been surgically unhinged was forced to walk by hospital staff. There seemed to be an inexplicably perverse belief that the more a symphysiotomy patient walked, the better. One mother described being forced to mobilise within a couple of days of her surgery at the Lourdes: 'they made me learn to walk up and down the stairs'. Walking further destabilised a pelvis adrift from its moorings, however.

Allegations of negligent care could also be levelled at general practitioners and public health nurses, who apparently did little to ensure adequate care. Public health nurses were supposed to visit newborn babies in the community within 24 hours of being notified of their birth.[294] Frequently, they examined the mother as well as the child.[295] And, under the Maternity and Infant Care Scheme, family doctors were required to examine the mother six weeks after the birth. Whether or not they were informed by hospitals of their patients' surgery is unclear, but how they could have failed to notice their walking difficulties is incomprehensible.

---

**13. Myths and red herrings**
'Excellent results were claimed for the procedure which permanently enlarged the pelvis and allowed women to have a normal delivery .... In properly conducted cases, complications were rare.' John Bonnar, Chairman of the Institute of Obstetricians and Gynaecologists, 2001.[296]

---

[292] Zhiyong Hou et al 2011 'Severe postpartum disruption of the pelvic ring: report of two cases and review of the literature' *Patient Safety in Surgery* 5:2. 3 Jan.

[293] R W Lindsey et al 1988 Separation of the symphysis pubis in association with childbearing A case report *Journal of Bone and Joint Surgery of America* 70: 289-92.

[294] TP Burke 1986 *Survey of the Workload of Public Health Nurses.* Institute of Community Health Nursing, Dublin, 26.

[295] Ibid, 9.

## A high risk operation

Symphysiotomy was described in 2010 as 'an alternative' to Caesarean section.[297] It was not an acceptable alternative, however. It represented the triumph of theology over reason. Almost all of the women who underwent these aberrant operations, and at least some of their children, suffered direct harm in consequence. Unlike Caesarean section, symphysiotomy and pubiotomy were widely known and reported both in Dublin and in Drogheda to be high risk. Pubiotomy was very widely seen as much more dangerous than symphysiotomy. A 1931 text enumerated its dangers: '1. The operation results in a compound fracture of the pelvis, therefore asepsis must be perfect. 2. Haemhorrage from the bladder veins. 3. Wounding of the bladder, and the formation of a fistula. 4. Wounding of the vagina.'[298]

Shaw's classic 1947 text gave a maternal mortality rate of 1.5 per cent for Caesarean section[299], far lower than some of the death rates quoted for symphysiotomy and pubiotomy in that era. A German review of pubiotomy had earlier quoted a fatality rate for mothers of 7 per cent.[300] Similarly high maternal death rates for symphysiotomy appeared in 1954, when symphysiotomy was at its height at NMH: Spanish doctors reported that ten women in a series of 259 operations had died from their genital wounds.[301]

The safety profile of the surgery in the literature was particularly poor for infants. High death rates were the norm. In the first half of the century, the mortality rate attributed to symphysiotomy was 9 per cent; rising to 11 per cent in the second half.[302] While these figures are not

---

[296] John Bonnar 2001 Letter to Dr Jim Kiely, Chief Medical Officer, Department of Health and Children. 4 May.

[297] John R McCarthy 2010 'Controversy over childbirth operation'. Letter *Irish Times* 1 March.

[298] Richard E Tottenham 1931 *A Handbook of Midwifery.* Churchill, London, 242.

[299] Wilfred Shaw 1947 op cit.

[300] A Schafli 1909 700 Hebosteotomien. *Z Geburtshilfe Gynakol* 64: 85–135.

[301] S Dexeus and N Salarich 1954. 'De la sinfisiotomia complementaria de recurso o de emergencia en el curso de la extraccion fetal por las vias naturales'. *Revista Espagnola de Obstetricia y Ginecologia* 13:358–366.

[302] Kenneth Bjorklund 2002 op cit.

scientific — because of the deficiencies of Bjorklund's review — they explain to a degree the suspicion that attached to the surgery within the specialty.

The risks for the mother were no less significant. These operations carrried a high risk of wounding to the bladder, for example, so urinary incontinence might have been expected. Instability of the pelvis would also, of itself, lead to a degree of incontinence. Complications of symphysiotomy reported in the medical literature apart from fatalities included incontinence and even fistula. Blood poisoning, inflammation of the abdominal lining, blood clotting, infection of the bone, rupture of the womb, inflammation, infection or abcess of the symphysis, abcess of the urinary tract, genital trauma, bruising or pooling of blood, walking difficulties, and pain in the symphysis, groin, hip, thigh and sacro-iliac joint, were among the complications documented.[303] Some of the surgery's dangers were graphically highlighted in South Africa by doctors who had experimented with the surgery at the University of Natal in Durban in the 1960s.[304] Seedat and Crichton underlined the importance of 'adhering to the midline' in severing the symphysis to prevent subsequent difficulties in walking. The Durban doctors were particularly critical of Zarate's technique which they felt might damage the sacro-iliac joint and lead to permanent pelvic instability and chronic pain, and recommended certain modifications.

Moreover, if one looks at these operations from outside the relatively narrow perspective of obstetrics, the inescapably problematic nature of the surgery becomes so apparent that no reasonable-minded person would contemplate its execution, except in an absolute emergency. Symphysiotomy severs a fused joint that is effectively the key point for stability in the body. The symphysis pubis is the mainstay of the pelvis, and the pelvis is integral to the structural and mechanical balance of the body. As well as supporting some of the main internal organs, such as the bowel and bladder, the pelvis also supports the spinal column.

---

[303] Ibid.
[304] D Crichton and E K Seedat 1963 'The technique of symphysiotomy'. *South African Medical Journal* 37:227–231.

Survivors have testified that the severing of the pelvis led to irreparable damage that the passage of time has intensified. Biomechanically, it would have been less destructive to break the femur, but such is the self-referencing power of obstetrics that it has succeeded in obscuring the inherently destructive nature of the surgery.

---

### 14. Myths and red herrings

'Nor would I defend the failures to give proper information to many patients, but such failures of communication were not confined to the obstetric section of the profession. Practice of 30 to 40 years ago cannot be judged by what is the norm today.' Dr Conor Carr, former Chairman of the Institute of Obstetricians and Gynaecologists, 2010.[305]

---

Access to contraception and to sterilisation would have solved the problems posed by repeat Caesareans, but these solutions were not offered. 'The doctors in question considered it a moral duty to ensure that women were not tempted to take what the doctors considered to be unethical decisions.'[306] They took it upon themselves to act as moral custodians to their female patients. None of the doctors involved in what Jacqueline Morrissey has termed 'the symphysiotomy experiment' proposed that information on birth control should be made available, even to 'high risk' women. Arthur Barry even objected to such information being given to NMH patients in 1963. Yet there was clear evidence of a demand for such information in the early 1940s. By denying women knowledge and by extension choice, doctors denied women the right to exercise their right to self determination Sterilisation was largely unavailable, if legal, due to doctors' objections.[307] So determined were they to ensure future childbearing unrestricted by contraceptive use that they gambled with their patients' health.

---

[305] Conor Carr 2010 'Symphysiotomy helped women have multiple births.' Letter *Irish Medical Times* 25 March
[306] Jacqueline K Morrisey 2004 op cit, 184.
[307] Ibid.

**Failure to inform the patient**

Obstetricians' failure to disclose relevant information to patients could also be seen to constitute negligence. The law requires a doctor to provide a patient with the information necessary to make an informed choice about treatment. Doctors already had a duty of care to inform the patient of such risks in 1944 and any suggestion to the contrary is baseless. The legal right to determine what shall be done with one's own body has been there for a hundred years.[308] Exercising that right requires knowledge. Failure to inform the patient of the risks of a particular intervention amounts to negligence.[309] Survivors of symphysiotomy have testified that, even at the level of information-giving, doctors failed in their duty of care towards their patients. Not one obstetrician, reportedly, informed his patient of the nature of the surgery she was about to undergo, the risks known to attach to the operation, the benefits attributed to it, or the existence of an alternative — and normative — treatment, namely, Caesarean section. Failure to disclose cannot be excused on the grounds that others engage in the same failure. These invasive operations were so egregious, their risks so real and foreseeable that no reasonably prudent doctor could fail to disclose them.

Moreover, the damage inflicted by the operation was damage about which the patient was entitled to be warned: in almost every case, at least some of the undisclosed risks that were known to attach to the surgery materialised. Those who habitually practiced these operations seemed to develop a blind spot that prevented them from foreseeing what any reasonably competent member of their specialty should have foreseen, based on what was known at the time about the surgery. The seriousness of the harm suffered by survivors is arguably testimony to the negligence exhibited by their obstetricians: prior to being operated upon, their victims were generally young, fit and healthy. Any woman, of any age or circumstance, would have needed to know the many material risks associated with these operations. Even if the risk was small, and there is no worthwhile evidence to suggest that it was, any reasonable person would regard such hazards as walking difficulties,

---

[308] John Seymour 2000 op cit, 203.
[309] ibid, 43-50.

chronic pain and urinary incontinence as significant. To deny a mother this information was to prevent her from exercising informed choice. Every competent human being has the right to determine what will be done with his or her own body, however. Exercising this right to autonomy depends on being able to make an informed choice. What woman, apprised of the nature of the operation and its dangers and knowing that a safer, universally accepted treatment was available, would have opted for the high risk and medically shunned practice of symphysiotomy?

### Surgery without consent

Survivors, without exception, have reported that these operations were carried out without their consent. The carrying out of surgery without consent has been unlawful for a hundred years.[310] Women were treated as inanimate objects of care, with doctors apparently relying upon the potentially abusive doctrine of assumed consent. In the only known instance of 'consent' being requested, permission was sought, not from the patient, but from her husband, although she herself was fully conscious and compos mentis at the time. Medical treatment requires direct consent, however, and this was surgery on a major bodily structure. The same abysmal failure to obtain consent in the 1940s and '50s persisted during the 1960s. Even in 1972, symphysiotomy was performed without consent on a patient at NMH,[311] and this flouting of patient autonomy continued into the 1980s.

While the law makes exceptions for emergency treatment, symphysiotomy was rarely performed on an emergency basis, as hospital reports show. Symphysiotomy were performed before a mother went into labour, in pregnancy or around the estimated date of delivery; in early or mid-labour; and in the aftermath of a Caesarean section. All were equally elective.

The law has long recognised a competent patient's right to decide what happens to his or her body. A pregnant woman is like any other competent adult: she has certain basic rights, such as the right to

---

[310] Ibid, 203.

[311] Marie Crean (her real name), personal communication.

decline medical treatment. This has been recognised for many decades at common law in the United States, Canada, England and Australia. The patient's right to autonomy was enunciated in the American courts as far back as 1914. In Schloendorff v Society of New York Hospital, for example, Judge Cardozo stated in his judgement: 'Every human being of adult years and sound mind has a right to determine what shall be done with his own body; and a surgeon who performs an operation without his patient's consent commits an assault, for which he is liable in damages.'[312] Dublin obstetricians appeared to be unfamiliar with the law. When Professor Ian Donald opined that patient preference, 'were she in full possession of all the medical facts', ought to be an 'acid test' for symphysiotomy, Arthur Barry responded by saying: 'surely it will be a sad day for obstetrics when we allow the patient to direct us as to the line of treatment which is best for the case.'[313]

Any intentional non-consensual touching that is harmful to a person's sense of dignity is actionable in law. Medical intervention that a patient has not consented to constitutes battery: the general rules that apply to battery are applicable to the doctor-patient relationship. Patients, where they are conscious and competent to make decisions, have the decisive role in medical decision-making. The right to determine what shall be done with one's own body is a fundamental right.

While the majority of symphysiotomies were carried out on patients who were conscious, some, such as those done before the onset of labour or in the aftermath of Caesarean section, were done under general anaesthetic. A small number of survivors have testified that they were asked to sign a 'blanket' consent form assenting to any operation the doctor might deem necessary. Such forms were in common use in Irish maternity units and hospitals. One consent form in use at the Lourdes Hospital in 1984 stated: 'I hereby give permission for the necessary operation and any additional work which may be considered advisable at the time, also I hereby consent and give permission for a General Anaesthetic on myself'. Another one, also in

---

[312] John Seymour 2000 op cit, 203.
[313] *Royal Academy of Medicine Transactions 1955 Irish Journal of Medical Science* 1955: 537. In Jacqueline K Morrisey 2004 op cit, 167-8.

use in that year, was similarly non-specific: 'I hereby consent and give permission for a General Anaesthetic and any operation the Surgeon considers advisable'.Even by the standards of the time, these forms were remarkably non-specific. Consent forms in Britain, for example, usually stated the purpose of the operation. In the absence of any information whatsoever about an operation so aberrant that it was unheard of, where the patient believed that the only possible operation that *could* be performed to deliver a baby was a Caesarean section — the signing of such forms by women could hardly be deemed to constitute consent.

To imply, as Dr Conor Carr has done, that it was acceptable '30 to 40 years ago' for a doctor to fail to give 'proper information' to a patient upon whom he was about to perform surgery is wrong. That failure — one that continued until the 1990s — was much more than a failure of 'communication': in the case of symphysiotomy, it effectively denied that patient her right to refuse that surgery. To carry out surgery without consent is illegal. Doctors' failure to obtain informed consent from the patient meant that the surgery constituted battery. The involuntary severing of the pelvis also breached women's constitutional rights, including the right to bodily integrity, the right to privacy, including self-determination, and the right to refuse medical care or treatment. In a 1996 case involving a person who had been made a ward of court, Judge Hamilton of the Supreme Court stated: 'the loss by an individual of his or her mental capacity does not result in any diminution of his or her personal rights recognised by the Constitution, including the right to life, the right to bodily integrity, the right to privacy, including self-determination, and the right to refuse medical care or treatment. The ward is entitled to have all these rights respected, defended, vindicated and protected from unjust attack and they are in no way lessened or diminished by reason of her incapacity. Judge Denham, also of the Supreme Court, stated: 'part of the right to privacy is the giving or refusing of consent to medical treatment ... As part and parcel of their constitutional rights, a patient has a right to choose whether she will or will not accept medical treatment. This concept is the requirement of consent to medical treatment seen from another aspect'.[314]

---

[314] Re A Ward of Court (No.2) [1996] 2 IR 79.

Moreoever, these symphysiotomies and pubiotomies were arguably a violation of internationally recognized human rights, viz., the European Convention on Human Rights of the Council of Europe,[315] which was based on the 1948 Universal Declaration of Human Rights. Article 5.1 of the 1950 Convention states: 'everyone has the right to liberty and security of person.' The Convention came into force for Ireland on 3 September 1953.[316]

## Unlawful medical experimentation

These operations were also unlawful if they were carried out for experimental purposes, because they did not meet the legal requirements for medical research. By 1947, these legal requirements had been codified in the Nuremberg Code. The revival of a long discarded operation at the National Maternity Hospital in 1944 was *de facto* experimental, as the unavailability of English language articles at the time on symphysiotomy and pubiotomy shows. One supporter of the surgery explained that mistakes were inevitable, because 'Dr Barry, Dr Spain and Dr Feeney are feeling their way with the new technique.' In 1949, defending one case of neonatal death and another case of Caesarean following symphysiotomy, Barry acknowledged the experimental nature of some of these surgeries. 'In extending the application of this operation, difficulties are bound to be encountered before the full limitations of the procedure can be appreciated.' Patients paid the price. Barry described a failed experiment — attacked by Professor Chassar Moir — where, 24 hours after the patient was admitted to NMH: 'Gross disproportion still existed, at this stage it was decided to submit the operation of symphysiotomy to as severe a test as possible. The symphysis was therefore divided...Twenty four hours later the head had descended almost to the level of the spines, but despite good contractions there was no advance. Profound foetal distress developed and lower segment Caesarean section was performed immediately. The head was deeply impacted in the pelvis and great difficulty was experienced in extracting the baby, which could not be revived.'[317]

---

[315] http://www.hri.org/docs/ECHR50.html.
[316] Ursula Kilkelly 2004 *ECHR and Irish Law*. Jordan, Bristol, lv.
[317] Arthur Barry 1950 *National Maternity Hospital Report 1950 Irish Journal of Medical Science* 1951:899. In Jacqueline K Morrisey 2004 op cit, 169–71.

Symphysiotomy was routinely performed at the Lourdes Hospital under circumstances so extreme that only an intention to test the operation to its limits could explain such outlandish clinical practice. The performance of surgery designed to deliver a baby on a woman who had just given birth by Caesarean section was difficult to comprehend on medical grounds, as the benefit to be derived by the patient from an unhinged pelvis was difficult to discern. Such a procedure may have been partly done for research purposes, to test whether or not symphysiotomy, carried out post Caesarean, would obviate the need for a repeat Caesarean in future births, and, if so, to establish in what percentage of cases. Operations performed prior to the onset of labour may also have been done to test the hypothesis that symphysiotomy performed at, say, 34 weeks could ensure a subsequent vaginal delivery, and, if so, in what proportion of births. Such surgeries could not be justified, say clinicans, on medical grounds. Some women had their pelvises measured before and after symphysiotomy; and, as in NMH, case histories were described in considerable detail.

Despite the liberal use of pelvic x-rays at the Lourdes (which would have led doctors in some cases to diagnose disproportion), there seems to have been a practice at the maternity unit of allowing some symphysiotomy patients to go over their due date. In 1962-63, for example, symphysiotomy was performed at 43 and 44 weeks; these babies were at the outer edge of postmaturity when placental disfunction may be lethal to the baby. The operation was also carried out in 1962-63 at 27 and 29 weeks, when fetal viability would have been unlikely. Only an intention to test the surgery at the outer limits gestation could explain such bizarre and dangerous practice.

Patient experimentation requires particular safeguards. In the traditional doctor-patient relationship, the patient trusts the doctor to act in his or her best interests, or at least, to do no harm, whereas in medical research, the doctor's primary goal may become the collection of data to the possible detriment of the individual patient. It is difficult to believe that Irish doctors operating after 1945/46 could have been unaware of the Nuremberg Code. The Nuremberg trials of Nazi doctors accused of conducting macabre human experiments in the concentration camps had received worldwide publicity, including in Ireland. Chief among these physicians was Dr Josef Mengele, who conducted 'genetic experiments' on nearly 1500 sets of twins at Auschwitz from 1943-44. Those subjected to his experiments did not know what his objectives were and his experiments, which included the removal of limbs and organs, were performed without anesthesia.[318] The Code was drawn up in August 1947 by the American judges who headed the trials and was the first of its kind to uphold the human rights of those subjected to medical research.[319] The Code emphasised, among other requirements, the absolute need to obtain the voluntary and informed consent of the person upon whom the experiment was being conducted. Another legal instrument that protected the human subject of medical research from the late 1960s was the UN International Covenant On Civil and Political Rights (1966). Article 7 states: 'No one shall be subjected without his free consent to medical or scientific experimentation.' While some symphysiotomies appear to have had an experimental dimension, no known safeguards were in place to protect the patient. And if there was experimentation, it was covert.

**Cruel and inhuman treatment.**
Seen from outside the perspective of obstetrics, these operations also assumed dimensions of extraordinary cruelty. As such, they were in breach of Article 3 of the 1950 European Convention on Human Rights, which says: 'No one shall be subjected to torture or to cruel, inhuman or degrading treatment or punishment.' In several cases, at least, the surgery was followed by sterility: survivors have testified that they found the entire experience so terrifying that they could never again bring themselves to have another child.

The cruelty of Zarate's method was striking[320]: it involved a partial incision of the symphysis, followed by the manual severing of the joint

---

[318] http://www.qcc.cuny.edu/socialsciences/ppecorino/MEDICAL_ETHICS_TEXT/ Chapter_7_Human_Experimentation/Case_Study_Josef_Mengele.htm.
[319]http://www.brown.edu/Courses/Bio_160/Projects2000/Ethics/THENUREMBURGCODE.html
[320] Mavis Kirkham, personal communication.

through the forcible splaying of the mother's thighs. There was also the cruelty of aberrant, and, possibly, experimental practice. In 1962-63, for example, one mother was allowed to carry her pregnancy to 44 weeks; before finally undergoing symphysiotomy, left in labour for 41 hours after her pelvis had been broken and was finally delivered by Caesarean section of a 10lb baby.[321]

Routinely carried out in the absence of medical necessity, all of these operations constituted cruel, inhuman and degrading treatment. Mothers selected for symphysiotomy were often obliged to labour for 24, 36, or 48 hours, to see if they could give birth without surgery, or to ensure that their cervixes had dilated sufficiently for the operation. Most were performed without prior notice. Women were unprepared for surgery and had no idea of what was being done. Their feet manacled, or held apart, their hands restrained, the symphysis was cut, or the bone sawn, and still they had to go on, for as long as it took, the pain of labour forcing its way through the agony of the surgery, until the baby came, and they could be delivered, by forceps, or by vacuum extractor.

These traumatic, invasive and agonising births were the norm in symphysiotomy and pubiotomy. Carried out, as they were, under the gaze of large numbers of doctors and midwives — all of whom must have known that Caesarean section was being withheld from the patient — these 'brutalising vaginal deliveries'[322] assumed Mengelian proportions.

There were degrees of cruelty. If the infant was in a particularly difficult position, such as a face presentation, giving birth with a broken pelvis was even more onerous. One mother described how her daughter was 'stuck for hours on end, in mid-cavity … The vein in my neck was swollen from pushing … You had to be awake, to push the baby into the world. It was a dreadful, dreadful experience'. To withhold Caesarean section from a mother whose baby was a brow presentation in the hope that it would convert into a face or a vertex presentation was

---

[321] *Our Lady of Lourdes Hospital Drogheda International Missionary Training Centre Clinical Report* Maternity Department 1962-63 op cit.
[322] Jacqueline K Morrisey 2004 op cit, 164.

cruel in the extreme. Yet, shockingly, both face and brow presentations seemed to be an indication for symphysiotomy at the Lourdes.

The widespread failure to give appropriate care after surgery led to a symphysis that failed to heal, or a bone that did not knit. The cruelty of performing surgery and failing to give proper post operative care was extreme. Mothers who tried, mistakenly, to walk in the aftermath of their surgery were not restrained, while some who attempted to remain in bed were forced to walk. Had the pelvis been kept stable at this time, the pain would have been considerably less. Measures that should have been taken, such as binders, were often neglected, reportedly, even in hospital. The same abysmal failure of care was seen in the community. General practitioners and public health nurses appear to have ignored the state of their patients, despite their evident inability to walk and their perceptible pain. Discharged without binders, without painkillers, without medical advice on the need for total bed rest; a complete ban on housework and childcare; and a long delay in sexual relations, women were left to sink or swim.

Finally, the logic of these operations, which were revived as a 'permanent cure' for disproportion, was troubling. Had the joint healed properly, or the bone knitted fully, then the permanent increase in pelvic diameter sought by doctors would have been improbable and, in particular, unlikely to have been sufficient to facilitate future vaginal births as intended. The success of the surgery was premised on the partial recovery of the patient.

# VII 'If they broke your pelvis': myths and realities

*You could only have three sections...But if they broke your pelvis, you could have nine or ten babies. That's what they wanted.*

Rosemary Harte, a survivor of symphysiotomy.

## Myths

### A totalising account

The totalising account of symphysiotomy first advanced by obstetrics since 1999 and subsequently adopted by senior cvil servants and successive Ministers for Health is one that portrays symphysiotomy as both necessary and appropriate, a life saver for mothers and babies alike for which 'excellent results' have been claimed. This homogeneising narrative, which is one of continuous progress in obstetrics, and successive advances, makes little reference to time, or place, virtually, and breaks down into two contradictory strands. The first is embedded in a view of symphysiotomy as the norm for obstructed labour until it was 'gradually replaced' by Caesarean section in the 1950s; while the second version acknowledges that Caesarean was the standard treatment, but presents symphysiotomy as a medical necessity in a pre-birth control era, performed to avoid the mortal dangers of repeat Caesarean section.

---

**15. Myths and red herrings**
'Maternal mortality was the main concern of all obstetricians in the 1940s and 1950s.' Peter Boylan and Tony Farmer, 1999.[323]

---

[323] Peter Boylan and Tony Farmer 1999 'Obstetrics and Ethics'. Letter *Irish Times* 6 Oct.

The IOG's 2001 presentation of symphysiotomy[324] is replete with errors. The view of a symphysiotomy as a norm for obstructed labour in Ireland until the 1960s is without foundation. Symphysiotomy failed to establish itself as a norm at any point in history, either in Ireland or anywhere else in the Western world, because it never succeeded in overcoming its dismal reputation as a risky procedure. Even today, its use in developing countries remains highly controversial. By the end of the 1930s, as has been demonstrated, Caesarean section was the procedure of choice for difficult births, even in Ireland, which was relatively slow to accept the new operation.

This narrative relies on 'shroud-waving',evoking the spectre of maternal death through the idea of a woman presenting in hospital in prolonged obstructed labour for whom a Caesarean, in the absence of antibiotics, might be fatal. This scenario appears to have been inspired by the annals of tropical literature: the IOG's letter gives a sense of this mother, exhausted and unfit to give birth, arriving on foot at the door of a hospital after several days' walking. Such a scene might have been credible in Famine times, but not in the Ireland of the 1940s. Symphysiotomy was not generally performed on an emergency basis. It was revived as an elective procedure, and this is borne out by hospital reports and medical debates, which overwhelmingly support survivor testimony on this point

This presentation also relies on the supposed frequency of maternal deaths from sepsis from 'about 1920 until 1960'[325], and relates them to the alleged non-availability of antibiotics. This is ahistorical: maternal mortality had fallen precipitously by the mid-1940s. The numbers of women dying from puerperal or childbed fever plummeted in Ireland in 1937,[326] as it did in Britain, even before the first sulphanamide drugs became available there in 1937.[327] The same dramatic drop in maternal

---

[324] John Bonnar 2001 Letter to Dr Jim Kiely, Chief Medical Officer, Department of Health and Children. 4 May.

[325] Ibid.

[326] Tony Farmar 1994 *Holles Street 1894-1994 The National Maternity Hospital–A Centenary History.* Farmar, Dublin, 107.

[327] L Colebrook and M Kenny 1936 'Treatment with prontosil of puerperal infections.' *Lancet* 5 Dec: 1319-26.

mortality was seen in mainland Europe and North America in the same year.[328] Sulphanamides were introduced to control infection in the main Dublin maternity hospitals in 1940.[329] Penicillin, first used in Holles St in 1944,[330] followed. The argument that maternal mortality was the main concern of all obstetricians in the 1940s and 1950s is therefore without foundation.

The further argument associated with this presentation — disputed by leading members of the IOG — is that symphysiotomy was done for pelvic disproportion at a time when cases of contracted pelvis were common. However, rickets, a 'deficiency disease' stemming from lack of vitamin D, sunlight and calcium[331] was rare. A brief spike in rickets was observed in small children — but not in pregnant women — in Dublin over the period 1941-3: poor quality flour was found to be the culprit and the problem was addressed without delay.[332] Rickets could not have been common, because it leads to a contracted pelvis; a contracted pelvis leads to disproportion and Holles St research showed that disproportion was an imaginary complication, as Dr Peter Boylan underlined.[333] This was the conclusion reached by Dr Kieran O'Driscoll,[334] who looked for evidence of disproportion in 1,500 first-time mothers. As he told the Royal Academy of Medicine in 1966: 'disproportion is a mote in the eye of the obstetrician - it does not exist.'[335]

---

[328] Marie O'Connor 1995 *Birth Tides*. Pandora, London, 10.
[329] Tony Farmar 1994 op cit, 52.
[330] Ibid, 120.
[331] Gladys B Carter 1939 *The Midwife's Dictionary and Encyclopaedia*. Faber and Faber, London.
[332] W J E Jessop 1950 *The Irish National Nutrition 1950 Survey Conference Proceedings*. Vol IV The Stationary Office, Dublin, 289-92.
[333] Peter Boylan and Tony Farmer 1999. Letter *Irish Times* 6 Oct.
[334] Kieran O'Driscoll, Declan Meagher with Peter Boylan 1993 *Active Management of Labor The Dublin Experience* 3rd ed. Mosby, London, 64-5.
[335] *Royal Academy of Medicine in Ireland Transactions 1966 Irish Journal of Medical Science* 1966: 570. In Jacqueline K Morrisey 2004 op cit, 187.

### 16. Myths and red herrings

'The obstetrician who responded to this problem [cephalopelvic disproportion] by doing a Caesarean section knew that he was probably condemning the woman to a large number of repeat Caesareans, with the risk to the mother's life as well as her health increasing with each succeeding operation.' Conor Carr, former Chairman of the Institute of Obstetricians and Gynaecologists, 2010.[336]

The second strand in the obstetric defence of symphysiotomy may admit that Caesarean section was the norm for obstructed labour, but justifies the surgery on the basis that it avoided the dangers of repeat Caesarean sections at a time when family planning was unknown. This apologia for symphysiotomy is as defective as the earlier one. To suggest that it was appropriate for doctors to subject women to the material and corporeal risks involved in severing the pelvis with a view to 'saving' them from the theoretical and statistical risks of repeat Caesareans is absurd. Also, the bald assertion that repeat Caesareans were dangerous hides the critical fact that, not only was vaginal birth after Caesarean permitted, but repeat Caesareans were common. The issue then becomes how many repeat Caesareans can safely be performed, but there was little ageement within obstetrics as to what constituted an upper safety limit. The infrequency of uterine rupture — one of the main complications of repeat Caesarean — in the main Dublin maternity hospitals in the 1940s suggests that the dangers of repeat Caesarean may have been inflated. The portrayal of symphysiotomy as a life saving operation depends on such exaggeration, however.

### 17. Myths and red herrings

'Because symphysiotomy permanently enlarged the pelvis the procedure also offered the prospect of safer vaginal delivery in future pregnancies at a time when large family size was usual.' Institute of Obstetricians and Gynaecologists, 2010.[337]

---

[336] Conor Carr 2010 'Symphysiotomy helped women have multiple births.' Letter *Irish Medical Times* 25 March.

[337] Institute of Obstetricians and Gynaecologists of the Royal College of Physicians of Ireland 2010 'Statement on Symphysiotomy' 17 February.

The presentation of symphysiotomy as a life saving operation also relies heavily on the erroneous ssumption that women were unable or unwilling to practice family limitation. This theory is not one that can be upheld over four decades of sustained symphysiotomy practice. Census data from the 1940s to the 1980s show that childbearing was not an immutable fact of life. To characterise even the 1940s — never mind the 1960s — as a pre-birth control era is wrong. Family limitation has never been synonymous with the use of artifical contraception. Abstinence was widely practiced as a method of family limitation.[338] By 1943 in Dublin, by whatever means, some women were planning their families.[339] Hysterectomy post Caesarean as a form of sterilisation appears to have been an established medical practice in Dublin by 1949.[340] Nor is there any evidence to suggest that Catholic working class mothers were particularly opposed to birth control, contrary to what has been claimed.[341] The Church's view on family limitation was not quite as monolithic as has been suggested. Pius XII authorised the use of the safe period in 1951.[342] By 1965, the Vatican Council had decreed that married couples should themselves decide when to have children and how many. By then, NMH had established the first family planning clinic for married couples in Ireland, while, by 1967, Holles St was offering 'the Pill' to those who felt 'in conscience' able to take it.[343] Oral contraceptives were widely prescribed as a 'cycle regulator'.[344] By the early 1970s in Dublin, family planning was widely available to married and unmarried alike. By 1973, despite *Humanae Vitae*'s condemnation of artificial birth control, over 20 000 women in Ireland were taking oral contraceptives.[345] And still the practice of symphysiotomy continued.

[338] John S Haller and Robin M Haller 1974 *The Physician and Sexuality in Victorian America* University of Illinois Press, Chicago, 125.

[339] Tony Farmar 1994 op cit, 116.

[340] Alex Spain 1949. 'Symphysiotomy and pubiotomy. An apologia based on the study of 41 cases'. *Journal of Obstetrics and Gynaecology of the British Empire* 56:576-85.

[341] Peter Boylan and Tony Farmer 1999 op cit.

[342] Tony Farmar 1994 op cit, 152.

[343] Ibid, 152-3.

[344] Maureen Harding Clark 2006 *The Lourdes Hospital Inquiry An Inquiry into peripartum hysterectomy at Our Lady of Lourdes Hospital Drogheda Report of Judge Maureen Harding Clark SC.* Stationary Office, Dublin, 251.

[345] Keith Wilson-Davis 1974 'The contraceptive situation in the Irish Republic'. *Journal of Biosocial Science* 6: 483-492.

The contention that symphysiotomy was performed to avoid the dangers of repeat Caesarean is embedded in a profoundly paternalistic view that denies women their autonomy. Dr John Cunningham, a former Master of NMH and close ally of John Charles McQuaid clarified where the locus of power lay: 'I do not consider that doing three Caesarean sections on a young women and then sterilising her is good obstetrics, nor is the wish of the patient an indication for sterilisation.'[346] The risk of repeat Caesarean section was one that intimately concerned the mother, one that could not be determined without her participation, or meaningfully evaluated except in the context of her particular circumstances. Dr Kieran O'Driscolls'[347] oft-repeated[348, 349, 350] assertion that symphysiotomy was performed *to offset the medical commitment* to repeat Caesarean is ultimately one that legitimises the abusive use of authority by consultant obstetricians who abrogated to themselves the right to impose a surgical, albeit potentially crippling, 'solution.'

# Realities

That such a dangerous and discredited operation as symphysiotomy could have been performed for upto five decades on over 1,500 women in hospitals across the state requires an explanation.

### The might of organised medicine

The practice of symphysiotomy was a reflection of the wider power relations in society, and, in particular, of the might of organised medicine, which predated the state by five centuries. Surgeons, for

---

[346] *Royal Academy of Medicine Transactions 1950 Irish Journal of Medical Science* 1950: 863. In Jacqueline K Morrisey 2004 op cit, 163.
[347] Kieran O Driscoll, Declan Meagher with Peter Boylan 1993 op cit, 65.
[348] Peter Boylan and Tony Farmer 1999 op cit.
[349] John R McCarthy 2010 'Controversy over childbirth operation.' Letter *Irish Times* March 1.
[350] Conor Carr 2010 'Symphysiotomy helped women have multiple births.' Letter *Irish Medical Times* 25 March.
[351] Marie O'Connor 2007 *Emergency - Irish hospitals in chaos.* Gill and Macmillan, Dublin, 81.

example, traced their roots to barber-surgeons who were first incorporated as a trade guild by Henry VI in 1446.[351] Around them grew some of the first so-called voluntary or private hospitals. Many, if not all, of these institutions were religious. Over time, these private hospitals came to constitute a significant power block over which the state sought to exercise little control. This was part of a wider pattern. A laissez faire attitude prevailed towards the reformatories, industrial schools, private orphanages,[352] county homes, Magdalen laundries, and mother and baby homes that were controlled by religious orders. The state's failure to protect patients mirrored its neglect of those incarcerated in these institutions. Private hospitals, such as the Lourdes, which embodied the power of the Catholic Church as well as that of institutional medicine, were generally allowed to run themselves, as the Harding Clark Report shows. Lack of state oversight of these hospitals partly explains how 800 or more of these aberrant operations could have been carried out, unquestioned, in three of these private institutions.

During the 50-odd years of its ownership by the nuns, the Lourdes Hospital was permitted to run its own affairs, unmonitored and unhindered. No state inspectors came to trouble the staff, or to examine the records. (The state inspection of hospitals was, and remains, reserved for public psychiatric inpatient facilities.) The operation of symphysiotomy was described and quantified in detail in clinical reports that were sent to both the Department of Health, the Royals College of Obstetricians and Gynaecologists in London and the Institute of Obstetricians and Gynaecologists in Dublin. Both the IOG, and its former parent, the RCOG approved of the maternity unit for training purposes.[353] The colleges asked no questions, apparently. Other authorities, such as the Nursing Board, also turned a blind eye. The same blind eye was turned towards the widespread practice of symphysiotomy at NMH and the Coombe Hospital, where such operations were similarly described and quantified in hospital reports that were sent to the same medical bodies.

---

[352] Eoin O'Sullivan and Mary Raftery 1999 *Suffer the Little Children The Inside Story of Ireland's Industrial Schools.* New Island, Dublin.
[353] Maureen Harding Clark 2006 op cit, 298.

The power of medical consultants, both within the hospital system and within the health service more widely, was another key factor. The approach to hospital management was described as 'command and control' by the Nursing Commission, which characterised management as 'quasi-militaristic' as well as hierarchical.[354] This view was later borne out by a professor of surgery, who described medical consultants as 'five-star generals'.[355] The lowly position of midwives within this medical army also helps to explain the lack of challenge to the practice of symphysiotomy.

**A culture of intervention**
The growth of obstetrics fostered a culture of intervention in childbirth. The Harding Clark Report paints a vivid picture of a hyper-medicalised system of maternity care run riot, where evidence-based practice was uncommon and patients were evidently at risk. High rates of induction, episiotomy and Caesarean section were the norm at the Lourdes Hospital, while the use of obsolete techniques, such as the disfiguring vertical incisions employed in the classic Caesarean section, seemed to be routine. Outcomes at the maternity unit were sub-optimal, with high infant mortality rates around the time of birth, and, in earlier decades, high death rates for mothers.

The culture of intervention in childbirth reached its apeotheosis in 1963 with the invention of a new regime in the labour ward. The real problem with women having their first baby, Dr Kieran O'Driscoll maintained, was not disproportion, it was 'inefficient uterine action'.[356] O'Driscoll proposed a new way of dealing with women's inefficiency in giving birth: the 'active management' of labour, a system that accelerated throughput in the delivery unit at a time when the hospital suffered from overcrowding. The 'new obstetrics' was grounded in 1950s authoritarianism, and required women to submit willy-nilly to invasive and painful interventions designed to speed up labour. Without

---

[354] Commission on Nursing 1998 *Report of the Commission on Nursing: a blueprint for the future.* The Stationary Office, Dublin, 137.
[355] Muiris FitzGerald 2002. In Ray Kinsella 2003. *Acute Healthcare in Transition in Ireland: change cutbacks and challenges.* Oaktree Press, Dublin, 57.
[356] Kieran O'Driscoll, Declan Meagher with Peter Boylan 1993 op cit.

its repressive culture, it is doubtful if women could have been symphysiotomised, as they were, without their knowledge or consent, up to 1984 and beyond.

## Gender inequality

The new system copperfastened the lowly position of mdwives within the hierarchy, leaving them effectively without clinical autonomy. Such a hierarchical system could be seen to militate against a sense of personal engagement and clinical responsibility. It led to professional silence, which led to patient endangerment, with midwives overseeing the aberrant practice of symphysiotomy in their labour wards for over four decades without demur, apparently. Even the presence of midwifery schools in NMH, the Coombe and the Lourdes, which must have provided some opportunity, however limited, for questioning abnormal practice in the labour ward, did not lead to the exposure of the surgery. In the Lourdes Hospital, for example, trainee obstetricians told the Harding Clark tribunal they feared for their careers, while midwives said they feared for their jobs. The dominant culture was one of collegial, if collusive, loyalty, underpinned by fear.

There was an element of gender inequality, as all midwives (and their 'patients') were female, while almost all consultant obstetricians of the era were male. It could be argued that midwives cared for their mothers as best they could, that they had been taught to defer to consultant opinion on issues of clinical practice. But, like medical trainees, midwives knew that Caesarean section was the norm for obstructed labour. Moreover, they were the specialists in normal birth: unlike obstetric students, they knew exactly how labour should proceed, and, within the midwifery model of care, it could be argued that midwives had a special duty of care towards the mothers under their tutelage. That they appeared to be unable to exercise this duty of care, even in the 1970s and '80s is a reflection of the hierarchical, managerialist straitjacket within which they worked. This straitjacket was further underlined by their failure to care for mothers appropriately post operatively. All midwives, in that era, had been trained as nurses: how to care for a broken pelvis must have been within their competence, but it was a competence they failed to exercise.

**The role of Catholic belief systems**

That the practice of symphysiotomy was impelled by personal belief systems is beyond doubt. Dr Alex Spain clarified the thinking that underpinned the surgery: 'the obstetrician is the man who should stand by whilst nature is fulfilled *per vias naturales* [by the natural route]. When he resorts to Caesarean section he has failed to stand by and how often also, outside Catholic communities, does he go further and destroy by mutilation [sterilisation] one of nature's most important functions?'[357] One mother attributed her doctor's failure to do a Caesarean to the fact that the Lourdes was a Catholic hospital: 'you were only allowed to have three Caesarean sections, so [if you resorted to birth control] you were curbing your family [and this was forbidden]'. Like other forms of birth control, such as sterilisation, the contraceptive pill was strictly prohibited at the Lourdes.

The chairman of the Irish Catholic Doctors' Association, consultant obstetrician and Professor Emeritus Eamon O'Dwyer has publicly stated that symphysiotomy was performed in Ireland for religious reasons.[358] It can hardly be entirely coincidental that the three hospitals that specialised in symphysiotomy, NMH, the Coombe and the Lourdes, were all under the control of Catholic Archdioceses. In hospitals where consultant contracts and ethics committees forbade practices such as artificial contraception and sterilisation, the operation of Caesarean section was bound to be viewed with some disapproval. The nexus of cross-relationships that existed included Archbishop John Charles McQuaid and leading Catholic obstetricians — all devotees of symphysiotomy — some of whom were members of prominent Catholic Action organisations — as well as the Medical Missionaries of Mary. The Archbishop of Dublin and chaplain of Holles St Hospital displayed a steely determination to control women's reproductive thinking as well as their health services. Part of the Church's role, as McQuaid saw it, was 'to determine and to control the social attitudes

---

[357] Royal Academy of Medicine Transactions 1950 op cit, 859. In Jacqueline K Morrissey 2004 op cit, 161.
[358] Karen Rice 2010 *Irish Daily Mail* 20 March.

of the family in the Republic, especially in the 'delicate' matters of maternity and sexuality.'[359]

## A natalist's dream

Symphysiotomy offered a surgical solution to the delicate matters of maternity and sexuality. The view of symphysiotomy as a mechanism to enable unlimited childbearing was borne out by Judge Maureen Harding Clark: 'Women seemed happy to have large families and symphysiotomy was carried out to facilitate this end.'[360] The report presented no evidence for the view that women wanted many children, however, and survivor testimony indicates that it was doctors who seemed happy for women to have large families, nine or ten children being the number that obstetricians encouraged them to have after breaking their pelvises.

The hostility to contraception and sterilisation shown by leading revivalists, such as Alex Spain and Arthur Barry, is a matter of record. So far as the practice of symphysiotomy was concerned, it is imposible not to conclude that doctors were playing God. Theirs was a body of knowledge rooted in medical texts of the 18th century, which portrayed women as incompetent;[361] theirs a legacy from the Victorian era, when brain studies 'demonstrated' women's intellectual inferiority[362] and it was no longer enough to be a minister of healing; one was also required to become a custodian of morals. Theirs was a perspective that saw Caesarean section as a barrier to Catholic family ideals, with women as vessels for making babies, and procreation the proper purpose of sexual relations within marriage. In carrying out a Caesarean section, however, doctors were effectively limiting the number of children that could be born to a woman.

Symphysiotomy was a natalist's dream; a gateway to the birth of babies as yet unconceived. The performance of symphysiotomy *after* a baby

---

[359] John Cooney 1999 *John Charles McQuaid Ruler of Catholic Ireland.* O'Brien Press, Dublin 259.
[360] Maureen Harding Clark 2006 op cit, 162.
[361] Jo Murphy Lawless Reading 1998 *Reading Birth and Death A History of Obstetric Thinking.* Cork University Press, Cork.
[362] John S Haller and Robin M Haller 1974 op cit.

was born is an indication of just how far some doctors were prepared to go to avert the 'moral hazard' posed by Caesarean section. Caesarean symphysiotomy was common at the Lourdes until 1970, and at least three such cases were carried out at NMH 'to overcome difficulties in future pregnancies'.[363] So it was not that women were endlessly falling pregnant, it was that doctors sought to avoid any procedure that might prevent them from doing so.

**The Africa connection**
Symphyisotomy also fulfilled other medical and religious ambitions. By 1944, the surgery had become a specialty of tropical medicine, as has been shown, offering a low cost alternative to Caesarean section in resource poor countries. NMH trained doctors bound for Africa and India from the 1940s onwards. The Lourdes Hospital was established to train medical missionaries for work overseas. Symphysiotomy was evidently taught there: one mother describes how 'there were 17 or 18 staff in the theatre ... There were anaesthetists, midwifery students, midwives, assistant gynaecologists, nurses'. Several of them were Medical Missionaries of Mary. Traffic from Ireland to Africa and from Africa to Ireland was strong. By the mid-1950s, well over 50 per cent of the medical personnel operating in Nigeria were Irish-trained, according to one member of the order working there in 1954.[364]

Outside Ireland, symphysiotomy has been almost exclusively reported in Africa from 1950-1999.[365] The surgery is viewed in many parts of the subcontinent as an operation that is performed only 'by white doctors on black patients'.[366] Many of the doctors who published articles on symphysiotomy in the medical press belonged to the colonising classes, to judge from their European surnames. From 1950 onwards, the

---

[363] 'NMH Report 1954' *Irish Journal of Medical Science* 1955:13. In Jacqueline K Morrisey 2004 op cit, 173.

[364] Margaret Mary Nolan 1954 'Obstetrical problems in Nigeria' *Irish Journal of Medical Science* May 341: 205-11.

[365] Kenneth Bjorklund 2002 'Minimally invasive surgery for obstructed labour: a review of symphysiotomy during the twentieth century (including 5000 cases)'. *British Journal of Obstetrics and Gynaecology* 109 (3): 236-48.

[366] Roeland Voorhoeve 2008 'Symphysiotomy – essential or obsolete?' *Bulletin of the Netherlands Society of Tropical Medicine and International Health* Dec 46 (6): 8.

operation of symphysiotomy was described in Nigeria, the Congo, Rhodesia, Tanzania, Uganda, Kenya, Zambia, Zaire, Malawi, Botswana and South Africa.[367] While NMH is credited by a former Master with transporting the surgery to Africa,[368] it would be a mistake to overlook the role of the Lourdes Hospital, as the widespread practice of symphysiotomy at the hospital owned by the Medical Missionaries of Mary in Afikpo, Ebonyi State, Nigeria shows.[369]

The symphysiotomy experiment at NMH has been described in considerable detail by Jacqueline Morrissey. Much of what passed for therapeutic symphysiotomy in the obstetrics department of the Lourdes Hospital also appeared to be of an experimental nature, as the persistence of the surgery for 20 years after it had been officially discontinued at NMH suggests. Sometimes it seemed that experimentation and teaching may have gone hand in hand. Josephine Lawlor's operation was performed six weeks before the birth: she recalled seeing a camera in the theatre before the general anaesthetic took effect. The deviant nature of some of these operations coupled with the minuteness of their documentation suggests that their primary objective may have been related, not to the clinical needs of the individual mother, but to the research and development requirements of the surgery. Four decades of clinical practice at the Lourdes resulted in a considerable body of data on symphysiotomy. The only evident beneficiaries were the Medical Missionaries of Mary and their burgeoning clinics and hospitals overseas.

**Women's powerlessness**
Women's powerlessness, both as life givers and as health professionals, lies at the heart of the symphyisotomy scandal, as one mother underlined: 'nobody questioned it. Nobody said, wait, can you do a section? It was their argument against yours, but you don't know ... The way you were treated, you didn't need to know'. Symphysiotomy

---

[367] Kenneth Bjorklund 2002 op cit.
[368] Kieran O Driscoll, Declan Meagher with Peter Boylan 1993 op cit, 65.
[369] IM Sunday-Adeoye, P Okonta and D Twomey 2004 'Symphysiotomy at the Mater Misericordiae Hospital Afikpo, Ebonyi State of Nigeria (1982-1999): a review of 1013 cases'. *Journal of Obstetrics and Gynaecology* Jan 24 (5): 525-529.

was driven, not by medical necessity, but by a reluctance on the part of certain male obstetricians to limit women's childbearing. For over four decades, without let or hindrance from the state, these Catholic doctors elected, willy-nilly, to sever women's pelvises in childbirth, eschewing a far safer operation, Caesarean section. A pitiless exercise in male medical power over female childbearing, symphysiotomy was a product of patriarchy, Western biomedicine, clericalism and colonialism. As well as lying four square with the prevailing natalist ideologies of the time, the surgery also served institutional needs, such as training medical staff for poorer countries, and, perhaps, perfecting the operation for missionary hospitals and clinics.

# VIII 'Before I go to my grave': a quest for justice

*They are waiting for us to die. I'd like to know why they did it, before I go to my grave.*

Rita Hartigan a survivor of symphysiotomy in Cork

Symphysiotomy is widely seen as the second biggest health care scandal in Ireland, the first being the contamination of the national blood transfusion supply, which resulted in the infection of over 3 000 casualties of the Blood Board with Hepatitis C and HIV. The widespread practice of symphyisotomy and pubiotomy at a time when Caesarean section offered an infinitely safer alternative raises troubling questions. Yet survivors' access to benefits and entitlements is a postcode lottery, they are statute barred from taking legal action and all attempts to secure an independent inquiry have been thwarted,

## Benefits and entitlements

The long term consquences of symphysiotomy reported by survivors are complex and wide ranging in some cases. A pelvis that has been unstable for three or four decades, for example, requires specialised care. Essential medical needs, such as effective pain relief, are not even being met in some of these cases. A comprehensive, integrated, specialised approach to survivors' healthcare is needed, one that reflects the fact that no two women have the same needs. Greater recognition — and reimbursement — of complementary therapies, for example, which some women find effective for pain relief, is required.

Ensuring women's access to appropriate and comprehensive health care, free of charge, is a priority. SoS medical cards that are 'for life' are urgently required: these cards carry a special patient identifier to enable the fast-tracking of hospital appointments, and the provision of items not on the General Medical Services list. Reimbursement for services, such as chiropody, physiotherapy, and osteopathy, to name but three, should be automatic. Home help needs to be brought up to a level commensurate with individual need. Continence supplies are also an issue: the bureaucracy that impedes reimbursement needs to be eliminated and choice of product should be available to all.

General practitoners have a critical role to play in ensuring women's access to appropriate health care, free of charge. An accurate information leaflet aimed at family doctors and pharmacists, prepared in conjunction with SoS, would help to inform general practitioners about symphysiotomy and its side effects. Also, liaison officers need to be designated in all areas of the HSE. These officers play a key role in ensuring women's access to services, negotiating the complexities of the system, and referring them to medical specialists and other healthcare practitioners as required. Finally, house renovations or modifications are a significant issue for the more disabled. Aids, such as stair lifts and walk-in showers, are urgently needed in some cases and, again, liaison officers can help to expedite matters with local authorities.

**The statute of limitations**
The statute of limitations, which requires the litigating of a complaint by an injured patient, for example, within two years of the date of knowledge of the event believed to have caused the injury, acts as a potent barrier to redress. In these cases, symphysiotomy was performed almost in a clandestine manner, with survivors denied all information by their caregivers prior to surgery and, in very many cases, following it. Justice demands that the statute be set aside for one year, to enable survivors to attempt to secure redress.

**Smokescreens**
Symphyisotomy remains uninvestigated, largely due to the smokescreens erected by the Institute of Obstetricians and Gynaecologists. The Murphy Report on clerical sexual abuse[370] showed that the need to protect the institutional Church took precedence over

---

[370] Yvonne Murphy, Ita Mangan and Hugh O'Neill 2009 *Commission of Investigation Report into the Catholic Archdiocese of Dublin Parts I and II.* July The Stationary Office, Dublin.

the imperative to protect innocent young people from priestly paedophiles. In this instance, the need to protect the specialty of obstetrics and gynaecology appears to have taken precedence over the moral imperatives of truth and justice. For over a decade, leading IOG members have sought to defend these operations to the hilt, while the Institute itself has engaged in a sustained endeavour to obscure the truth. There has been no accountability, only denial; no transparency, only obfuscation.

The triumph of collegiality over justice continues. The IOG's 2001 letter to the Department of Health falsely conjuring symphysiotomy as a norm for obstructed labour in the period from 1944 has been used repeatedly to torpedo all endeavours to secure an independent inquiry. Following the *Prime Time* programme, the external review promised by the government in 2003 was reduced to the status of an internal report from a private body with a vested interest. Indeed, Mary Harney's request to the IOG appeared to have been framed in the Institute's own constructs. Those same terms have now been given to a historian from University College Cork, who, following consultation with the institute[371] has been commissioned to undertake a report on the surgery by the Minister for Health. No requirement flows from these terms of reference to answer critical questions, such as why the operation was exhumed, or why it was performed instead of Caesarean section.

Whether or not the report writing team originally assembled by the IOG, which included an obstetrician who headed an initiative overseas teaching skills that included symphysiotomy remains in place is unclear. Whether or not the Institute's plan to review the tropical literature on symphyisotomy is going ahead is also unclear. Such a review would frame the practice of symphysiotomy in Ireland in the context of medicine in Africa; and there is some indication that this may yet be done, as the report commissioned from University College Cork is to examine 'the Irish experience relative to other countries'.[372] Such a

---

[371] Jennifer Martin 2011 Email to Tom Moran 12 May
[372] Danielle Barron 2011 'Symphysiotomy report to be carried out'. *Irish Medical News* 23 May.

requirement brings with it a risk that the pro-symphysiotomy bias inherent in the tropical literature on the surgery may yet find its way into an official report.

There seems to be no intention to assess the surgery's side effects among survivors. The long-term safety of the operation has yet to be established,[373] however, and almost all the Irish evidence is to the contrary. Irish survivors offer a golden opportunity to pursue research that is of global significance. The long term safety of a once obsolete operation now being mainstreamed in resource-poor countries should now be evaluated.

**A vested interest**
The latterday practice of symphysiotomy was an abusive use of medical authority. Had the government left it to the Irish Hierarchy to investigate allegations of diocesan sexual abuse, there would have been a public outcry. Yet the Department of Health continues to look to the IOG, a body with a vested interest in showing symphysiotomy in a positive light, for guidance in this matter. Describing the IOG's 2001 report as ' contemptuous', Senator David Norris told the Senate the Institute was 'not fit to be charged with this [issue]'.[374] Symphysiotomy, he said, 'was not a matter of one or two operations. It was a deliberate and consistent practice, which was known and ignored by the professional body, and now we are sending it back to them'.

The hypothesis that symphysiotomy may have been carried out, at least partly, for training purposes is not a line of inquiry that can be expected from any official report. Both the Institute and the RCOG likely validated the operation for training purposes for decades, in a country where no evident need for such training existed. Moreover, it was IOG/RCOG members who carried out, authorised, ordered, supervised, or were otherwise responsible for these operations. Those who did not themselves perform the surgery work in hospitals where these operations were executed, on a very significant scale in the

---

[373] G J Hofmeyr PM Shweni 2010 'Symphysiotomy for feto-pelvic disproportion'. Cochrane Database of Systematic Reviews 2010 Issue 10 30 Aug. John Wiley.
[374] David Norris 2010 *Seanad Debates* Order of Business. Vol 201 No 2 Col 59 4 Feb.

Lourdes, the National Maternity and the Coombe. In a culture where institutional loyalty is prized above all else, and professional collegiality has triumphed time and again over patient safety, such affiliations must give rise to grave concern among those who wish to see justice done. Litigation anxiety may also be a potent barrier to truth, as one Caesarean symphysiotomy case is currently before the courts.

**Patient safety**
Few meaningful safeguards to protect patients have reportedly been put in place in the Lourdes Hospital since the publication of the Harding Clarke Report in 2006. Nationally, there are no active proposals for an inspectorate for acute hospitals, while audit has yet to become an integral part of clinical practice. The proposed hospital licensing system has yet to be implemented and concern has been expressed that the system may rely on self-reporting and form-filling. Medical practice remains effectively unmonitored, hospital risk management is suboptimal, quality assurance mechanisms are lacking and meaningful peer review has yet to be developed.

Changing structures in the health system are expected to lead to a further shrinking of accountability. Health legislation enacted since the abuses at the Lourdes maternity unit came to light denies citizens an entitlement to an independent hearing. The 2004 Health Act removed from patients a right they previously exercised, namely, the right to bring complaints involving medical treatment to the hospital in question or to a public health authority. Patients are now obliged to take such compaints to the Medical Council, a body with a long tradition of not investigating such matters. Indeed, the Harding Clark Report, by proposing that patient records be exempt from freedom of information legislation, did little to promote transparency and accountability.

Ireland is not a particularly safe country in which to have a baby. Several of the major health scandals in Ireland in recent years, such as the forced sterilisations at the Lourdes Hospital, or the recent antenatal scans misdiagnoses, have occurred in obstetrics. The high medical intervention rates that characterised the Lourdes Hospital are the norm almost everywhere. Caesarean section rates stood at 26 per cent, nationally, in 2009[375]: such a hyper-medicalised system is leading to poor outcomes. Ireland's infant death rates in or around the time of birth continue to be among the highest in the European Union. In 2006, for example, only some of the former Eastern bloc countries, such as Romania, Bulgaria and Latvia, showed significantly higher infant death rates around the time of birth.[376] Up to 200 babies are diagnosed every year with cerebral palsy[377] : some have been shown in court to be casualties of oxytocin, the synthetic hormone that is a cornerstone of the active management of labour.

While symphysiotomy is no longer practised, the same warped and gendered power relations that enabled these abusive operations to be carried out are still in evidence. Survivor Nuala Kavanagh underlined the gender aspect: 'a man wouldn't do it to a man, but a man would do it to a woman, [and] a vet would probably not do it to an animal'.Around 75,000 women have a baby in Ireland every year under conditions that are effectively determined by a very small private body, comprising 125 members[378] or so, the vast majority of whom are male. Maternity care policy has been frozen since 1976. The old hospital hierarchies are still largely in place, while the active management of labour, itself a quasi-militaristic system, is more prevalent than ever. The legal and ethical requirement to seek informed consent, so widely ignored over more than four decades of symphysiotomy, continues to be flouted. In a national survey of maternity care in 2008, 58 per cent of respondents said they were denied the right to refuse medical intervention.[379] As hospital services become more centralised, the need to get women through the bottle-neck of the labour ward in the shortest possible time may take precedence over the requirement to respect their autonomy.

[375] Niamh Healy, personal communication. See www.bump2babe.ie/column/P/statistics

[376] Economic and Social Research Institute 2008 *Perinatal Statistics Report 2006* Health Research and Information Division December. ESRI, Dublin, 9.

[377] Marie O'Connor 2007 *Emergency - Irish Hospitals in Chaos* Gill and Macmillan, Dublin, 61.

[378] Institute of Obstetricians and Gynaecologists 2006. *The Future of Maternity and Gynaecology Servces in Ireland 2006-2016* Report from Institute Subgroup December. Institute of Obstetricians and Gynaecologists RCPI, Dublin, 11.

[379] Association for Improvements in the Maternity Services in Ireland 2008 *Report of a Survey on the Availability of Information and Consent.* March AIMS Ireland, Dublin.

This report suggests that the maternity care sector as a whole is in need of fundamental review. Symphysiotomy was, and is, a 'technology' of obstetrics. While Irish maternity care is based on obstetrics, the specialty of abnormal birth, other countries with superior systems of care, such as Germany and the Netherlands, give a far greater role to midwifery, the specialty of normal birth. Scientific evidence shows that midwifery-based care offers a safe, cost effective, service.[380] The development of new structures of maternity care, however, has been impeded by the IOG, whose opposition to midwifery-based care can hardly be unrelated to the market for private obstetrics, which in 2004 was estimated at €49m.[381] Private fees have increased significantly since then.

**The public interest**
Allowing such a profound breach of doctor-patient trust to go unexamined corrodes public confidence in the health service as a whole. The State's continuing refusal to investigate this aberrant surgery is not only denying survivors justice and truth, but it is also denying the caring professions and the health system at large an opportunity to learn from some of its most salient failures. As Frances Fitzgerald, now Minister for Children, told the Senate in 2010, 'it is critical that we learn lessons about why these procedures were carried out and the principles that determined they be undertaken because, clearly, they were not medical.'[382] While the carrying out of symphysiotomy as an operation of last resort under conditions where Caesarean section is unavailable may be life saving, those circumstances did not apply to these operations, which were performed alongside Caesarean section. The Ireland of 1944 was not a society that was ill served by modern medical facilities.

The failure of the medical profession to learn from its travails has been conspicuous, not unlike that of the Catholic Church. Three decades of

---

[380] Declan Devane et al 2010 *A systematic review, meta-analysis, meta-synthesis and economic analysis of midwife-led models of care.* Royal College of Midwives, London.

[381] Marie O'Connor 2006 In Andrew Symon 2006 Ed. *Risk and Choice in Maternity Care An International Perspective.* Churchhill Livinsgtone Elsevier, Edinburgh, 110.

[382] Frances Fitzgerald 2010 *Seanad Debates* Order of Business. Vol 201 No 2 Col 54 24 Feb.

forced sterilisations at the Lourdes was dismissed as 'a systems failure' by the editor of the Irish Medical Journal.[383] One of the three consultant obstetricians who exonerated Michael Neary was subsequently elected President of the Royal College of Physicians in Ireland (the parent body of the IOG).

No known process has ever been instituted against the medical consultants, the doctors in training, the midwives and the nurses who acquiesced for three decades with the involuntary sterilisations at the Lourdes Hospital. None of the professional bodies responsible for standards in the various specialties took any formal steps, apparently, to investigate their members' conduct. These bodies, primarily the Institute of Obstetrics and Gynaecology, the Royal College of Physicians and the Royal College of Obstetrics and Gynaecology, but also the College of Anaesthesia, the Nursing Board and, to a lesser extent, the Irish College of General Practitioners, are also implicated in the practice of symphysiotomy.

The final indication of a failure to learn from these sorry chapters in maternity care comes from the Nurses and Midwives Bill 2010, which proposes to subordinate midwifery to nursing. If this is passed into law, then midwifery will be the sole regulated profession in health and social care in Ireland to be ruled by another profession. Patient safety demands that midwifery be given independence from nursing within governance structures that include appropriate lay representation. A more powerful midwifery profession might have blown the whistle earlier on the maverick practice of symphysiotomy and pubiotomy.

**Natural justice**
The responsibility of the State and its liability for the multiple and serious injuries sustained by symphysiotomy patients are beyond dispute. Symphysiotomy and pubiotomy may have been a product of patriarchy and clericalism that reflected the power of the medical

---

[383] J F A Murphy 2006 *The Lourdes Hospital inquiry: its implications for medical practice. Irish Medical Journal* 99 (3): 68-69.
[384] Institute of Obstetricians and Gynaecologists 2010 op cit.

profession and of the Catholic Church, but it was regulatory failure that allowed 1,500 or more of these grotesquely dangerous operations to be carried out, unquestioned, for up to five decades.

In their variety, complexity, gravity and longevity, the side effects of symphysiotomy reported by survivors today are comparable to those suffered by mothers who contracted Hepatitis C from infected blood. For some, symphysiotomy led to a lifetime of loss that may never be redeemed. Without an impartial and comprehensive study, however, the extent or severity of their injuries may never be known. The same observation can be made in relation to children born by symphysiotomy.

The widespread failure to give appropriate post operative care ensured the worst possible outcomes for patients. In severing the pelvis and neglecting to give post surgical care, consultant obstetricians were, in effective, maiming women. The same inexplicable failure to give appropriate care could be seen in the community among general practitioners and public health nurses. Failed by their hospitals, their obstetricians, their midwives, their family doctors, and their public health nurses, survivors were let down by an entire health system.

Survivor, Vera Kennedy points out that no one has ever taken responsibility for these operations. 'They should say: we now apologise because you are in pain and in grave discomfort.' The failure to admit wrongdoing has meant that no process of any kind has ever been initiated against those who carried out, condoned or facilitated these debilitating operations. All involved failed signally to protect their patients. The state's moral failure to take responsibility for these abuses by holding those responsible to account is equalled only by that of the Catholic Church in relation to clerical sexual abuse. The resignations by Irish bishops set a new standard for those in high positions, however. The logic of the Murphy Report and its aftermath suggests that consultant obstetricians who performed or were in any other way responsible for symphysiotomies, or who concealed or misrepresented these operations in recent years, should be relieved of all responsibility, direct and indirect, for patient safety.

Older women, many of them grandmothers, attribute the last government's failure to deal with the issue to their female gender, advancing age and increasing infirmity. Some have concluded that inertia has been chosen as the final solution; that the authorities, having stalled them since 2003, are waiting for them to die. Justice cries out against such a policy. Survivors' need for closure is imperative. They need to know why they were selected for symphysiotomy or pubiotomy; and why they were denied access to the standard treatment: Caesarean section. They need to know who was responsible for severing their pelvis, and why it was done in their particular case, as Teresa Moroney explains: 'I want the answers for my husband, for my children. I want them to know it was a wrong practice'. Survivors need to know why they were never told about the operation before or, often, after it was performed; why the risks were not explained; and why they were given no opportunity to decline such dangerous surgery. They need to be helped to get on with their lives. Rosemary Harte talks of the need for acceptance: 'there are people out there who know what happened. They have to set us free, they have to come forward'.

Those affected by these tragedies need an acknowledgement of wrongdoing: if there was negligence, if there was battery, they need those responsible held to account. They need redress for a lifetime of pain and suffering, a lifetime of missed occasions and blighted opportunities. For some, there is also the issue of lost children, of babies who did not survive the procedure, and sons and daughters they could never bring themselves to have, due to fear of childbirth post symphysiotomy. As they face old age, with its threat of increasing pain and mobility difficulties, they need answers. They need those answers before they go to their graves.

Only a truly independent and wide ranging inquiry will satisfy the demands of patient safety, the public interest and natural justice. Vera Kennedy summed it up: 'It shouldn't have been done. Caeserean sections were there at the time. It was bad doctoring ... You don't take a block out from the bottom of the house, because there's going to be cracking. The pelvis is the same, it's the foundation of the house'.

# Appendix 1 | IOG letter to CMO 2001

## The Institute of Obstetricians and Gynaecologists
### of
## The Royal College of Physicians of Ireland

Chairman          PROF. J. BONNAR        Patron:   MARY MCALEESE,,        6 Kildare Street, Dublin 2
Hon. Secretary:   DR. H. O'CONNOR                  President of Ireland    Telephone: 661 6677
Hon. Treasurer:   PROF. R. HARRISON                                       Fax: 676 3989
      04/05/01                                                    4th May 2001

Dr. Jim Kiely,
Chief Medical Officer,
Department of Health & Children,
Hawkins House,
Dublin 2.

### Re: Symphysiotomy

Dear Dr. Kiely,

Thank you for your letter of 25th April 2001 concerning recent publicity in the media about the use of symphysiotomy in obstetrical practice in the 1950s and '60s.

From about 1920 until 1960 operations of symphysiotomy were employed in selected cases in Dublin mainly in the National Maternity Hospital and the Coombe Hospital. Excellent results were claimed for the procedure which permanently enlarged the pelvis and allowed women have a normal delivery. This was a time when caesarean section did have a high mortality due to sepsis and the operation of symphysiotomy had the advantage of enlarging the pelvis and allowing the women to have subsequent normal deliveries. In properly conducted cases complications were rare. Spain (1949) reported 36 cases with no maternal deaths and Barry (1956) recorded a total of 165 cases without maternal death and an infant loss of 10. Feeney (1956) reported 114 cases without maternal death and infant loss of 11. Many of these cases were emergency admissions with obstructed labour where sepsis following caesarean section, would have carried a significant risk of maternal death. In these years sepsis was one of the leading causes of maternal death.

From 1950 onwards the operation of symphysiotomy for obstructed labour was replaced by the modern caesarean section; by then antibiotics were available to treat infection and sepsis became much less of a hazard.

I should mention that the operation of symphysiotomy remains an accepted indication for the management of a trapped after coming head of a breech. This again will become something in the past as caesarean section is now recommended for all mature infants who present with a breech presentation.

I enclose a copy of a chapter dealing with symphysiotomy by Professor John F Cunningham former Master of the National Maternity Hospital and Professor of Obstetrics and Gynaecology, University College Dublin, published in British Obstetric and Gynaecological Practice (1959), which contains the references I have given above.

Yours sincerely,

*John Bonnar*

Dr. John Bonnar,
Chairman,

John Bonnar 2001 Letter to Dr Jim Kiely, Chief Medical Officer,
Department of Health and Children. 4 May.

# Appendix 2 | The Bjorklund review

Bjorklund's 2002 review[385] of what he termed this 'minimally invasive surgery' was little more than a statistical mish-mash based on all the papers sourced by his researchers published on symphysiotomy during the 20th century. His literature review exposed major defects in the obstetric database, however.

Doctors' knowledge of symphyisiotomy was largely based on tiny, statistically insignificant studies. Criteria for inclusion in the Bjorklund review were extremely low by generally accepted statistical standards: papers used by him to calculate maternal and fetal mortality rates were based on as few as 25 cases, while other 'studies' used to calculate morbidity or sickness rates, such as the percentage of women who suffered a fistula following the surgery, were derived from patient numbers of 5-24. Bjorklund utilised these figures to produce aggregates and percentages of his own, seemingly unaware of, or, alternatively, ignoring the fact that just over 1000 cases are required for any *one* study to be considered fully statistically reliable.

Adding the results of invalid studies together to generate global statistics did not add value. On the contrary, such additions gave rise to even further problems, when like was not compared with like, and problems of definition were ignored. One doctor looked at women's walking difficulties on the seventh day following surgery, for example, while another counted cases where 'confident walking was delayed beyond four weeks'. Bjorklund saw no difficulty in adding 'walking difficulties' (plus or minus) at one week to 'confident walking' at one month and over to devise new aggregates and the walking difficulties themselves were undefined.

There were also problems of cultural bias. Extrapolating from the dead to the living was one difficulty: obstetrics, like other medical specialties,

---

[385] Kenneth Bjorklund 2002 'Minimally invasive surgery for obstructed labour: a review of symphysiotomy during the twentieth century (including 5000 cases)'. *British Journal of Obstetrics and Gynaecology* 109 (3): 236-48.

had come from just such a tradition. Another bias was evident from the fact that doctors had a tendency to underreport adverse outcomes, focusing on fetal deaths and ignoring fetal injuries, for instance. The medical perspective on what should be considered a bad outcome from the surgery was highly selective. Take sexual difficulties, for example. Such problems might reasonably have been expected following surgery that maimed the sexual organs. The Swedish doctor made only one reference to sex, however, quoting without comment a European doctor in Uganda in 1982, who pronounced that 'within a month most [symphysiotomy] patients have recovered sufficiently to undertake all family and marriage commitments'.

Bjorklund's work revealed, albeit unintentionally, that doctors had no idea of either the medium or long-term consequences of the surgery. Studying those consequences would have required particular effort, given the structure of maternity care. Postnatal care routinely picked up only on short-term problems, as doctors usually saw their patients for a final check six weeks after the birth.

Brorklund's work is of historical interest, however. From 1900-99, doctors studied the side effects of symphysiotomy in less than 500 women Only three long-term follow up studies of symphysiotomy were reported in the 20th century, all of them statistically worthless. The short term monitoring was little better. During the first half of the century, doctors reportedly tracked just 79 women for a period of days or weeks, while from 1950-99, doctors observed a total of 227 mothers, according to Bjorklund. He also revealed that follow up studies over a period of years were almost unknown, with obstetricians studying the long-term effects — variously defined — of their handiwork in just 129 women over a period of 100 years.

Ignoring the striking lack of good quality evidence from a century of what passed for research into the surgery, Bjorklund concluded: 'The results indicate that symphysiotomy is safe for the mother from a vital perspective, confers a permanent enlargement of the pelvis and facilitates vaginal delivery in future pregnancies, and is a life saving operation for the child. Severe complications are rare.'

Symphysiotomy, he further advised, should be reintroduced into the medical curriculum for use in 'Third World' countries. 'If valid conclusions can be drawn from one hundred years of retrospective studies, there is considerable evidence to support a reinstatement of symphysiotomy in the obstetric arsenal, for the benefit of women in obstructed labour and their offspring', he concluded, sweepingly.

It is upon Dr Bjorklund's utterly invalid article that the medical consensus that symphysiotomy is 'safe for mothers' rests.

Efforts to promote the low-cost operation in these countries are being led by a very small number of obstetricians in Northern Europe, who insist that symphysiotomy is safe for mothers. The operation has become extremely controversial in tropical medicine in recent years. Many obstetricians in Africa refuse to carry it out. The surgery is known to cause fistula, one of the biggest problems in maternal health in poorer countries. Swedish and other doctors have bemoaned the 'widespread resistance among obstetricians in the Third World' to the surgery.

# Appendix 3 | IOG Statement on Symphysiotomy

**'Statement on Symphysiotomy'**
Questions have been raised about the practice of symphysiotomy in Ireland. The Institute of Obstetricians and Gynaecologists, RCPI considers it important to express its position as regards the practice of the procedure.

Members of the Institute offer our unreserved sympathy and support to any mother who may have experienced complications following symphysiotomy.

The Institute has previously written in support of mothers who suffered adverse outcomes following the procedure. In these letters, the Institute has recommended that mothers should be given a full explanation, to which they were entitled, and that their grievances should be considered sympathetically.

The Institute fully supports HSE and Department of Health & Children initiatives to assist those who have suffered complications of the procedure.

The Institute recommends that data on symphysiotomy be incorporated into a National Clinical Audit on obstetric practice.

**What is surgical symphysiotomy?**
Symphysiotomy may occur spontaneously in late pregnancy or labour, or as a result of a surgical procedure. Surgical symphysiotomy is a procedure carried out on the pubic symphysis joint of the pelvis, under local or other anaesthesia.

The cartilage of the joint and some of the supporting ligaments are incised. This results in permanent widening of the pelvis by up to 3.5 cms. The joint heals with laying down of dense connective tissue.

The World Health Organisation includes the procedure in its coding manual International Statistical Classification of Diseases (ICD-9-CM Code 73.94).

**What are the benefits?**
The increase in pelvic size allows vaginal birth in selected cases of obstructed labour. This in turn reduces maternal and infant death and morbidity rates and complications such as urinary incontinence from vesico-vaginal fistulae that can result from prolonged obstructed labour.

The technique may also be used to aid delivery of the infant in births complicated by shoulder dystocia or entrapment of the after-coming head in breech delivery (see below).

**What are the complications?**
Immediate complications may include pelvic joint pain and difficulty walking. Bladder infection and incontinence may occur. There may be injury to local tissues with haematoma (bruising and clot) formation and local infection.

Reported long term problems include walking difficulties, pelvic joint pain and urinary incontinence. These may subside after 3 to 6 months (Bjorkland, 2002).

**Why was symphysiotomy used?**
The procedure was introduced in the 18th century for selected cases of obstructed labour and proved effective in allowing vaginal births while reducing maternal and infant death and morbidity rates that related to prolonged labour.

Because symphysiotomy permanently enlarged the pelvis the procedure also offered the prospect of safer vaginal delivery in future pregnancies at a time when large family size was usual.

At that time, symphysiotomy was a simpler and safer practice than caesarean section (C/S), a technique that gradually replaced it during the 20th century when difficulties with the C/S procedure itself were overcome. Caesarean birth, until the operation was refined, was itself a cause of maternal death, mainly due to blood loss and infection.

**Is symphysiotomy valid nowadays?**
In some countries symphysiotomy may still be used as a life saving procedure for the mother and infant in circumstances where caesarean section is technically not an option (Liljestrand, 2002; WHO, UNFPA, UNIEG, World Bank 2001).

The technique is no longer used in this country as an alternative to caesarean section for obstructed labour.

Exceptionally rare emergency situations may arise when the technique could be used such as (a) severe shoulder dystocia when, after the delivery of the head, the infant's shoulders cannot pass under the pubic symphysis, or (b) when a baby is being born as a 'breech' its head becomes trapped in the mother's pelvis.

In these situations, symphysiotomy may be considered as valid when a range of other obstetric interventions have failed.

The procedure does not form part of the Irish curriculum of specialist training. However, the technique is taught as an emergency procedure on the 'Management of Obstetric Emergencies and Trauma' course of the Royal College of Obstetricians and Gynaecologists, London which many Consultants and Trainees have attended.

The historic use of symphysiotomy should be assessed in the context of what was considered valid practice at the time. Medical research papers regarding symphysiotomy were produced from other countries at the time when the technique was being performed here.

## References

Bjorkland, K (2002) Minimally invasive surgery for obstructed labour; a review of symphysiotomy during the 20th century (including 5000 cases). BJOG, Vol, 109, pp 236-248

Liljestrand, J (2002) The value of symphysiotomy. BJOG, Vol, 109, pp. 225-226

'Managing Obstetric Emergencies and Trauma' (2007) Royal College of Obstetricians and Gynaecologists (RCOG), London

WHO, UNFPA, UNIEG, World Bank. (2001) Managing complications in pregnancy and childbirth. A guide for midwives and doctors. Geneva: WHO

Institute of Obstetricians and Gynaecologists of the Royal College of Physicians of Ireland 2010 'Statement on Symphysiotomy' 17 Feb.

# Appendix 4 | IOG Terms of Reference

## Symphysiotomy in the Republic of Ireland

### Terms of Reference

- Prepare a report on the practice of symphysiotomy, including a comparative analysis of the rates of the procedure, for the consideration of the Minister for Health and Children

- Meet with the group of women who underwent the procedure to gain more understanding of their experience and the impact it has had

- Assess the circumstances in which symphysiotomy was carried out in Irish Hospitals

- Determine the role of relevant professional bodies in guiding its members on guidelines, consent and monitoring its practice

- Detail when and why its place changed in clinical practice when it became significantly less prevalent

- To carry out a systematic review of all relevant literature about the place and effects of symphysiotomy

Institute of Obstetricians and Gynaecologists of the Royal College of Physicians of Ireland 2010 Terms of Reference.

# Appendix 5 | SoS Terms of Reference

1. To inquire into the clinical practice of symphysiotomy and pubiotomy in Irish hospitals and nursing homes from 1944 onwards, with particular reference to the reasons for the revival of the surgery, its subsequent proliferation, and relevant related issues;

2. To review and make findings on the management of care of all women and their children still living who underwent symphysiotomy and pubiotomy, or, where deceased, whose close relatives have come forward on their behalf, as to the appropriateness of the surgery and the adequacy of the medical services provided to them;

3. To reach conclusions and make recommendations to improve the conditions of women and their children still living who underwent symphysiotomy and pubiotomy;

4. To make such further or other recommendations as may arise from the inquiry to help to improve the conditions under which women give birth today in Irish maternity hospitals and units.

These terms of reference were proposed to the Chief Medical Officer at the Department of Health and Children on 25 August 2010.

SoS further stated 'that a formal inquiry, based on the above recommendations, should include, but not be limited to, the nature of these operations and their history, globally; the introduction and development of Caesarean section in Ireland; the reasons for the revival in Dublin of symphysiotomy and pubiotomy in 1944; the extent and duration of the surgery in Ireland; the reasons that impelled this widespread clinical practice; and whether or not symphysiotomy and pubiotomy served training and/or other institutional needs.'

'Case-by-case examination should include: the reasons for the surgery; the giving of patient information prior to surgery; the seeking of informed consent; the technique employed by the obstetrician; the clinical results, as evidenced by x-ray or other diagnostic tools; post-operative medical care in hospital and in the community; the outcomes, short, medium and long term, of the surgery; and continuing health and other needs in consequence of the operation.'